BACKCOUNTRY
FIRST AID
and Extended Care
Fourth Edition

by

Buck Tilton, M.S.

Director
Wilderness Medicine Institute of NOLS

Published by The Globe Pequot Press
Guilford, Connecticut

Dedication

This little book is dedicated with big love, deep respect, and infinite gratitude to my family, Melissa Gray and Zachary Gray Tilton.

Backcountry First Aid and Extended Care 4th edition

Copyright © 2002 by Buck Tilton

Illustrations by David Gross

Library of Congress Cataloging-in-Publication Data is available.

Manufactured in the United States of America

First Edition/First Printing

The author and publisher have made every effort to ensure the accuracy of the information in this book at press time. However, they cannot accept any responsibility for any loss, injury, or inconvenience resulting from the use of information contained in this guide. Readers are encouraged to seek medical help whenever possible. This book is no substitute for a doctor's advice.

Contents

List of Figures

Foreword

A medical emergency, when it occurs in the wilderness, can be a frightening experience—especially if someone else is the victim and you are the one who must provide care. There is no 911 to call nor paramedics who will arrive within five minutes. There's nothing but you and a patient in shock from a fall, a severed artery, or a rattlesnake bite.

An Emergency Medical Technician (EMT) would know what to do. He or she is no stranger to the first aid publications of Buck Tilton. They are likely to be one of the thousands of outdoor professionals who have graduated from one of the first aid courses that Buck offers at the Wilderness Medicine Institute of NOLS.

This edition of *Backcountry First Aid*, like all of Buck's books, is not just for the medical professional. It is for everyone who enjoys the outdoors. Even if you aren't an EMT, it will give you the knowledge and confidence to handle most injuries or illnesses that you may encounter. It will help you get over the shock of having to face a first aid emergency, teach you to assess the situation, and get you started on taking the right steps to properly treat and protect the patient from further harm.

It doesn't take a medical professional to understand the simple and straightforward presentation of Buck Tilton. The text reflects a mixture of common sense and best practices, within the context of the situation. His style is easy—comfortable and non-threatening. Read it and you will become part of Buck's following—not a fan, but a disciple—one who comes back for more—whether it's a refresher course or a new edition of this book. Read it and you will feel forever comfortable, wherever your outdoor experience takes you.

1: Introduction

Time is the essential element distinguishing first aid from extended care. When the doctor is far away, an hour or more according to the Wilderness Medical Society, the principles of first aid are often unequal to the task of managing the injured and the ill. And consider the rough trail, the wandering length of river, or the long miles of black asphalt separating the patient from a medical facility. Think about the heat or cold, the rain, the wind, the darkness. Remember that equipment needed for treatment and evacuation may have to be improvised from what is available. Remote locations and harsh environments may require creative treatments. All these things are the stuff of extended care.

It is the responsibility of those who live and work in isolated places to have the ability to act appropriately in an emergency. Like all talents, first aid and extended care can be learned. Excellent opportunities to gain the knowledge and practical skills were few and far between not long ago. Now they are available regularly in many communities. This booklet does not pretend to have all the answers. It provides principles for dealing with many serious emergencies and a few common problems. It is intended to be a reminder about what to do for those who have training and a stimulus to learn for those who are untrained. It is not intended to be a substitute for professional medical care when such care is available.

2: Action Checklist

1. Take a deep breath. **Stay Calm. Take Charge.** Be quick but not hasty. **Act fast—but go slow.**
2. Make sure the **Scene is Safe.**
3. Perform an **Initial Assessment**, treating the patient for any immediate threats to life or limb.
4. Perform a **Focused Exam and History**, examining the patient of any injuries, gathering information, assessing the patient's stability.
5. Sit down, relax, and **Plan What To Do**. Treatment must be considered and carried out, an evacuation may need to be prepared, help may need to be requested.
6. **Stay or Go, Fast or Slow.** If an evacuation of the patient is necessary, decide if you need to move quickly or at a more leisurely pace.
7. Keep a **Written Record** of the emergency.
8. **Act** in the best interest of the most people.

3: First on the Scene

Leadership

When an emergency arises, there is seldom time for democracy (let's-take-a-vote) or laissez-faire (what-will-be-will-be) leadership. The situation requires a kindly autocrat, someone who takes charge, a benevolent monarch demanding the greatest good for the greatest number.

A leader needs to see the whole picture. Though a leader's medical skills may be great, they are often best utilized by telling others what to do. By standing back, a leader can see everyone and everything and make sure nothing is left undone.

Leadership at an emergency should be calm and methodical. Calmness may be the most important ingredient in a successful rescue. Act calm and, after a while, you may actually start to feel calm. Quick action and hasty action are not the same thing. Haste makes waste, and sometimes the waste is of human life or limb. Act fast—but go slow. Every situation differs, but knowing a sequence of events that will work in an emergency can provide a powerful foundation for proper care (*See Action Checklist*).

Size-Up the Scene

During a rescue, you must do all you can to insure you **never create a second patient**. Make sure the scene is safe. Humans are resources who can think, help tend the patient, participate in carrying a litter. A second patient not only doubles the trouble, but also reduces the resources—the problem is more than twice as serious. Precious moments taken to stand apart and survey the scene for safety are often the most valuable of the rescue.

1. Are there immediate dangers to rescuers or patient, e.g., rockfall, avalanche, lightning?
2. What is the safest route to use approaching the patient?
3. Are there subtle dangers involved for rescuers or patient, e.g., chill, wind, heat?
4. Can anything be done to make the scene safer?

Initial Assessment

Your goal in the Initial Assessment is to identify and treat any immediate threats to life. Immediate loss of life will be from: 1) loss of **Airway**, or 2) inadequate **Breathing**, or 3) loss of adequate **Circulation** because the heart has stopped or too much of the patient's blood is in the wrong place, e.g., on the ground, spilled inside a body cavity, 4) extensive **Disability** from damage to the cervical spine, or 5) **Exposure** to environmental extremes, e.g., intense cold. Once safely at your patient's side, check the ABCDEs.

Airway

An airway starts at the nose and mouth and ends deep in the chest where oxygen is exchanged for carbon dioxide. If it's not open all the way, it won't work.

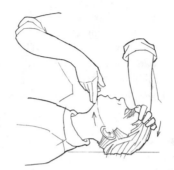

Figure 1: Head Tilt-Chin Lift

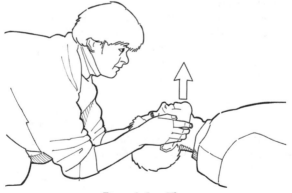

Figure 2: Jaw Thrust

In an unconscious patient, the most common airway obstructions are the back of the tongue and the epiglottis. By tilting the head back and lifting the chin—the head tilt-chin lift maneuver—most airways can be opened. If a spine injury is suspected (*see Spine Injuries*), use the jaw thrust maneuver, a maneuver that does not endanger the spinal cord, to open the patient's airway.

In a conscious patient, food is the most common obstruction. If he or she can speak or cough, do nothing but watch and wait. If the patient goes silent or starts to wheeze, it's time to give Dr. Heimlich's maneuver a try: Stand behind the patient and wrap your arms around him or her with one hand formed into a fist and pressed into the patient's abdomen, thumb side of fist in, just above the navel. Cup your fist with your second hand. Pull in and up with a quick, forceful motion. If the object is not expelled, repeat the maneuver until it works. (**Note**: You can perform the Heimlich Maneuver on yourself if you find yourself alone and choking.) For patients who are very pregnant or very obese, wrap your arms around the chest with your fists pressed into the sternum (breastbone), and perform the same thrusting motion.

If the patient goes unconscious before the airway is cleared, lower him or her gently to the ground. Open the mouth and look in to see if there is an object you can observe and remove. Open the airway with a head tilt-chin lift. If breathing does not immediately start, attempt a ventilation by pinching the nose closed, sealing your mouth over his or her mouth, and attempting to blow air into the patient. If the attempt fails, reposition the patient's head and try again. If no air goes in, perform 15 chest

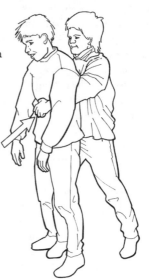

Figure 3: Heimlich Maneuver

compressions as you would do in CPR *(see below)*. Then open the mouth wide in order to see if any obstructions have become visible. If obstructions are visible, remove them. Attempt ventilations again *(see above)*. Keep up this sequence until the airway is cleared.

Note: Any rescue breathing is a safer bet in terms of your personal health and well-being if you use a pocket rescue mask.

If you find a patient who appears unconscious, check immediately for responsiveness by a gentle shake and a shout: "Are you OK?" If he or she does not respond, open the airway and place your ear near the mouth to **Look**, **Listen**, and **Feel** for air movement. If the patient is breathing, continue with the Initial Assessment. If no breathing can be detected, attempt to give the patient a rescue breath. If your air won't go in, reposition the head and try again. If air still won't go in, perform 15 chest compressions as you would do in CPR *(see below)*. Attempt ventilations once again *(see above)*. Continue this sequence until the airway is cleared.

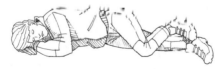

Figure 4: Recovery Position

Breathing

If your check for breathing reveals no respiratory activity, and your ventilations go in, and the chest rises as you breath in showing that air is getting into the lungs, that means the patient has an adequate airway but is not using it. You must keep breathing for this person.

After two initial full breaths, pause long enough to check for a heart beat. A beating heart will be indicated by breathing, coughing, movement, and/or a pulse. To check for a pulse, place two or three of your fingers over the carotid artery, in the valley between the windpipe and the large neck muscle, just below the angle of the jaw. If you find indications of a beating heart, continue rescue breathing by giving one ventilation approximately every five seconds. (If the patient is a child, give breaths faster—about once every four seconds.)

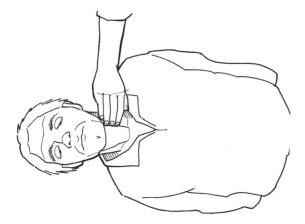

Figure 5: Checking the Carotid Pulse

Circulation

Rescue breathing, remember, is useless if the patient does not have a beating heart to push around the blood you're oxygenating with your breath, Cardiopulmonary resuscitation (CPR) is presented briefly here, but remember: CPR needs to be seen and practiced to be learned well. CPR courses are offered regularly by either the American Heart Association or the American Red Cross in most communities.

19

Note: If you do not have a rescue mask and you do wish to perform mouth-to-mouth ventilations, at least perform the chest compressions.

CPR: *One Rescuer*
1. Assess responsiveness with a gentle shake and a shout.
2. Turn patient onto back, if necessary, while supporting the head and neck.
3. Open the airway (head tilt-chin lift) and assess breathing (look, listen, feel).
4. If no breathing is evident, give two slow full ventilations, watching for the chest to rise and allowing it to passively relax between breaths.
5. Check for signs of a beating heart: breathing, coughing, movement, and/or a pulse.
6. In the absence of signs of a heart beat, begin chest compressions by placing one hand on the middle of the sternum at approximately nipple level, placing your other hand over the first, keeping your arms straight, and pressing down 1.5 to two inches. Depress the sternum 15 times at a rate of 100 compressions per minute.
7. After every 15 compressions, give two slow full ventilations.
8. After four cycles of 15:2 (approximately one minute), recheck for signs of a beating heart. If no signs are found, continue the cycles of 15 chest compressions to two breaths.

Note: Any patient with adequate breathing and circulation, either before or after CPR, should be rolled into the recovery position to insure maintenance of the airway.

Bleeding

Life-threatening arterial bleeding pulses or spurts from a wound each time the patient's heart beats. Venous bleeding, which can also be serious, flows smoothly and rapidly.

A quick visual scan of the patient is often enough to detect serious bleeding—but not always! Check inside the clothing of someone wearing bulky winter gear or rain gear. Check beneath someone who is lying in sand, rocks, or any terrain that might disguise blood loss. Severe blood loss can also be internal (see Shock).

To control any bleeding, apply pressure from your hand directly on the wound. If the wound is on an arm or leg, elevate the injury above the level of the patient's heart to reduce blood flow even more.

Note: Before contacting blood, or any other body fluid, the safest bet in terms of maintaining your own health is to wear protective gloves. If there is a chance blood could be splashed into your eyes, wear glasses, e.g., sunglasses.

If blood loss is tremendous, and death imminent, a tourniquet can be used on an arm or leg. Improper use of a tourniquet, however, may lead to loss of limb. Tie a band of material, preferably three to four inches wide, around the limb, as close to the wound as possible but above the elbow or knee, and snug it down until blood loss stops. Loosen it slowly after approximately 10 minutes to see if clots have closed the wound. Re-tighten the tourniquet if you need to, but leave it in place no longer than necessary.

Serious wounds should be splinted after the bleeding has stopped in order to prevent excess movement that might restart the blood loss (see Musculoskeletal Injuries, Splinting).

Disability

Down through the vertebrae (backbones) runs the all-important spinal cord. If its nerve messages are impeded by damage, the result may be permanent paralysis or death. In the initial phase of treatment, any patient who might have a spine injury, especially a cervical (neck) injury, should be kept still with calm words and hands on the head until secondary treatment can be applied (see Spine Injuries).

Highly suspect injuries include:

1. Those that leave the patient unconscious.
2. Those that are produced by potentially neck-breaking mechanisms such as sudden forceful stops, falls from a height, and diving from a height accidents.
3. Those that cause the patient to complain of neck and/or back pain.
4. Those that produce tenderness in the neck and/or back (it hurts when you touch there).
5. Those that produce altered sensations in the extremities (tingling, numbness, the inability to move hands or feet).

Exposure

Prolonged exposure to environmental extremes can cause changes in body core temperature that threaten the patient's health. For that reason, a patient should be protected from the environment, e.g., gently placed on a sleeping pad and covered to protect from cold, as soon as safely possible. "Exposure" also reminds you that you must sometimes expose parts of the patient's body in order to assess the extent of damage.

Focused Exam and History

The Focused Exam and History is a complete field examination of the patient. Its goal is to find everything that is not in perfect working order. It includes three phases, but they seldom fit into neat little groups of things to do. The three phases are presented here that way for simplicity. In the end, you want to make sure you've overlooked nothing relating the patient's well-being.

Patient Exam

Check the patient from head to toe in order to find any damaged parts. **Look** for wounds, swelling or other deformities, removing clothing if necessary. **Ask** where it hurts, and if it hurts when touched. **Feel** gently but firmly, a massage-like action with your hands spread wide to elicit a pain response but without causing further damage. Be aware of unusual smells (e.g., alcohol) or sounds (e.g., labored breathing). If you suspect an injury may be hidden beneath clothing, you must take a look at skin level. "Go to skin to assess" is the mantra of the rescuer.

Check:

1. Head, looking for depressions in the skull, damage to the eyes, fluid in the ears or nose or mouth.
2. Neck, for pain or deformity.
3. Shoulders, for pain and symmetry with the other shoulder.
4. Chest, for ability to take a deep breath, uneven breathing movements of the chest wall, abnormal breathing sounds.
5. Abdomen, gently pressing for pain or abnormal lumps.
6. Pelvis, by pushing on the two pelvic crests.
7. Back, by reaching under the lower back of someone on his or her back. If the patient is on her side when you find her, check the back before rolling.
8. Genitals, if it seems relevant.
9. Legs, including symmetry and the ability to move the feet.
10. Arms, including symmetry and the ability to move the hands.
11. After a head-to-toe check, carefully roll the patient found flat on his back in order to fully assess the back (*see Spine Injuries*).

Vital Signs

Vital Signs are measurements of the physiological processes necessary for normal functioning. They do not tell you what is wrong, but they do tell you how the patient is doing. Changes in vital signs over time are indicators of changes in the condition of your patient. Check early, and keep checking. To better monitor a patient, record the time at which you take a set of vitals. Signs include:

Level of Consciousness: A prime indicator, a check on how well the brain is communicating with the outside world. Use the AVPU scale for quick reference.

(A)   Is the patient **Alert**, able to answer questions?

A+Ox4: Patient knows who, where, when, and what happened? Note: If the patient knows what happened, he usually knows the rest of the story as well.

A+Ox3: Patient cannot remember what happened but does remember who, where and when.

A+Ox2: Patient can only relate who and where.

A+Ox1: Patient only remembers who he is.

(V)   Does she or he respond only to **Verbal** stimuli? Grimacing or rolling away, for instance, from your voice when you speak or shout? In what way does the patient respond?

(P)   Does she or he respond only to **Painful** stimuli, such as a pinch? In what way does the patient respond?

(U)   Is she or he **Unresponsive**?

Skin: Normal skin is pink (in non-pigmented areas such as the inner surface of the eyelids and the fingernail beds), warm, and apparently dry to your touch.

Heart Rate: Count the number of heartbeats per minute. For speed, count for 15 seconds and multiply by four. Note the quality of the pulse. Is it weak or strong, regular or irregular? Normal heart rates are strong and regular, and somewhere between 50 and 100 beats per minute.

Breathing Rate: Count the number of breaths per minute without telling the patient what you're doing. If she knows you're checking, she typically alters her breathing rate in an attempt to be accommodating. Normal lungs work about 12–20 times per minute at any easy, regular pace.

Note: Without a watch, you should still get a rough estimate of rates. Rough guesses are better than no idea.

Patient Interview: The History

More information is usually gathered by subjective questioning that by objective checking. Hopefully, the patient will provide the answers. Sometimes witnesses are sources of important information. Ask calmly, and do not use leading questions, e.g., say "Describe your pain" instead of "Is it a sharp pain?" Be aware of your tone of voice, your body language, eye contact. Patients usually feel better and respond better if they think you're really nice—but don't make promises you can't keep. If you gain trust, you must maintain trust.

The SAMPLE Questions:

S for **Symptoms:** Pain, nausea, lightheadedness, other things you can't see.

A for **Allergies:** Any known allergic reactions? What happens?

M for **Medications:** Anything legal or illegal? Why?

P for **Pertinent Medical History:** Anything like this happen before? Currently under a physician's care for anything?

L for **Last Intake and Output:** When was food or drink last taken? How much? When was the most recent urination and defecation? Were they normal?

E for **Events:** What led up to the accident or illness? Why did it happen?

S.O.A.P.

In an emergency, your brain tends to become a sieve instead of a bowl. The acronym SOAP reminds you to write everything down as soon as possible—as long as taking notes doesn't interfere with patient care. Retention of information for medical and legal reasons is important.

S for **Subjective information:** who, how, where, when, and what the patient complains of.

O for **Objective information:** vital signs, results of patient exam, results of patient interview.

A for **Assessment:** what you think is wrong.

P for **Plan:** what you're going to do.

(A) for Anticipated Problems: how might the patient change over time?

4: Shock

Shock is a condition that results when the body's cells are not getting a sufficient flow of adequately oxygenated blood. It can occur from a great variety of injuries and illnesses including blood loss, dehydration, heart attack, spinal cord damage, and a severe allergic reaction.

Whatever the cause, shock patients share similar signs and symptoms: Level of Consciousness is one of anxiety and restlessness that may progress to unconsciousness and coma. Heart Rates increase and grow weaker. Breathing Rates increase and become shallower. Skin usually turns pale, cool and sweaty. Thirst and nausea are common complaints.

Whatever the cause, shock can kill! Backcountry treatment for shock is limited. Early recognition and management are critical. At first, **assume shock in all patients until it is proven otherwise.** Shock patients who do not soon stabilize and start to improve—monitor the vital signs—need rapid evacuation.

Treatment for Shock
1. Secure and maintain an airway.
2. If a cause can be identified, such as bleeding, treat the cause.
3. Keep the patient calm and reassured.
4. Keep the patient lying down and protected from loss of body heat.
5. Elevate the patient's feet approximately 10 to 12 inches,

or place the patient on terrain with the feet slightly higher than the head.

6. Although food and drink are not usually recommended, small sips of cool water may be given to prevent dehydration on a long evacuation. The patient must be able to accept and drink from a container.

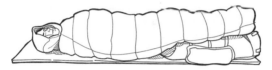

Figure 6: Shock Treatment Position

Evacuation Guideline
Evacuate any patient who exhibits signs of sustained or progressive deterioration.

5: Spine Injuries

The first goal of spine injury management is to prevent any further injury. To accomplish this, the patient's spine needs to be immobilized and stabilized. If the patient has suffered a highly suspect injury (*see First on the Scene, Initial Survey, Disability*), he or she must be initially immobilized by keeping him or her still and with a pair of rescuing hands on the patient's head. A patient found unconscious should be considered spine-injured until proven otherwise.

Process for Clearing the Spine

1. Complete a full patient assessment (*see First on the Scene*). To clear the spine, you must have a fully reliable patient: at least A+Ox3 on the AVPU scale, sober, and without distractions such as severely painful injuries or deep psychological distress.
2. Check a second time for reliability.
3. Check a second time for altered sensations in the extremities: tingling, numbness, weakness, inability to move. To clear the spine, you must have a patient with no altered sensations in the extremities.
4. Fully and carefully press on all the bones of the neck and back a second time. To clear the spine, you must have a patient who is free of pain and tenderness in the spine.

Managing the Spine-Injured Patient

A patient whose spine cannot be cleared has a broken back until proven otherwise. When the spine-injured patient has to be moved, say into a tent for warmth or out of an avalanche zone, move him or her via Body Elevation And Movement (BEAM). Get as many hands on the patient as possible, with firm ones on the head. At the command of the head-holder, lift the patient **as a unit** with as little spine movement as possible, and carefully carry him or her to a pre-designated spot.

A patient on his or her side can be log rolled onto the back. Manual stabilization of the neck is critical during the roll. At the command of the head-holder, the patient is rolled **as a unit**. A log roll can also be used to roll a patient onto his or her side in order to place a pad underneath before rolling the patient back onto the pad.

If the patient's neck lies at an odd angle, it may be straightened with very gentle support and slow movement to line it up with the rest of the spine. If this movement causes pain or meets resistance, stop and immobilize the patient's head as it lies.

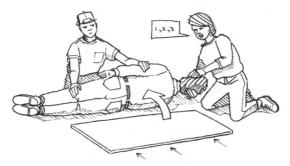

Figure 7: Log Roll

With the spine in normal alignment, the next step is to stabilize the cervical spine. Ambulances carry rigid cervical collars. You can improvise one in the backcountry with a SAM Splint®, extra clothing, or by cutting off the end of foamlite sleeping pad to fit the patient's neck and taping it in place.

31

Collars, even commercial products, do not totally stabilize the cervical spine. Hands-on attention should still be maintained, if possible, until the whole patient is stabilized in a rigid litter. In the backcountry, you're often looking at a long wait for a litter, but attempting to move a spine-injured patient without one creates great risk and is not recommended. When a litter is available, the patient should be FOAMed in place—made Free of Any Movement—with lots of padding and straps. Avoid the voids with pads under the knees, in the small of the back, and anywhere there's space that could let the patient shift. The patient's head should always be strapped down last. Proceed with care: Permanent spinal injuries often result from improper handling in the field.

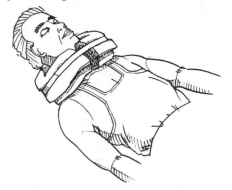

Figure 8: Improvising a Cervical Collar

Evacuation Guideline
Evacuate anyone being treated for spinal injury.

6: Head Injuries

Head injuries—and here we're talking about trauma to the brain—can be loosely divided into two categories:

Mild Head Injury

Despite the possibility of heavy bleeding from a scalp wound or the growth of a goose-egg sized bump, serious damage is rare if the skull is intact and the brain relatively undamaged. The patient may have lost consciousness but responded immediately to aggressive stimulation: loud shouts, forceful pinches. Treat wounds appropriately: Pressure from a bulky dressing on the bleeding scalp, and a cold pack for the bump. Keep an eye on the patient for about 24 hours. Awaken the patient every couple of hours during the night to check on level of consciousness (*see below*).

Severe Head Injury

Unconsciousness in which the patient does not respond to aggressive stimulation may indicate serious brain damage. Move the patient carefully and check carefully for cervical spine damage that is sometimes associated with a severe blow to the head. Keep the patient lying down. If possible, elevate the head and shoulders slightly. Do not give pain medications. If breathing becomes erratic or slow and labored, start rescue breathing. Rapid evacuation will be necessary if there is any indication of a skull fracture.

Signs of a Skull Fracture
1. A depression in the skull
2. A visible fracture where the scalp has been torn away.
3. Bruising around both eyes (raccoon eyes) or behind both ears (Battle's Sign).
4. Cerebrospinal fluid sometimes mixed with blood weeping from nose or ears.

Signs of Obvious Brain Injury
Head-injured patients may appear OK, and then start to deteriorate. If any of these signs or symptoms show up, immediate evacuation is required:
1. Level of consciousness deteriorates from disoriented to irritable to combative to coma.
2. Heart rate slows down and bounds.
3. Respiratory rate is erratic, or slow and labored.
4. Skin becomes flushed and warm, especially the face.
5. Pupils become distinctly unequal.
6. Protracted vomiting.
7. Visual disturbances.
8. Seizures.
9. Increasing and severe headache.

Evacuation Guideline
Evacuate anyone with signs and symptoms of severe head injury. Evacuate anyone who does not respond

initially to aggressive attempts at stimulation after a blow to the head.

7: Chest Injuries

Any injury to the chest may lead to respiratory difficulty and a critical patient. A simple fractured rib (*see Fractures*) may not be so simple if a bone fragment punctures a lung. Air escaping the lung and collecting in the chest is called a **pneumothorax** with increasing difficulty breathing and a rising level of anxiety. A pneumothorax can worsen until the patient is unable to breathe adequately, a condition known as a **tension pneumothorax,** which may result in death. Suspicion of a pneumothorax calls for an immediate evacuation.

If several ribs are broken in several places, a free-floating section of chest wall, called a **flail,** often results. The flail will move in opposition to the rest of the chest wall during breathing. This condition is extremely serious. Taping a bulky dressing over the flail may allow the patient to breathe a little more easily. The tape should not be placed entirely around the chest, a technique that makes it more difficult to breathe. During the rapid evacuation—the speed of which may be all that saves the patient's life—the patient may require rescue breathing. Evacuation of the patient on his or her side, injured side down, sometimes aids breathing.

If the chest has been opened by a penetrating object, the hole may bubble and make noise when the patient breathes. This is called a **sucking chest wound**, and the hole should be immediately covered with an occlusive dressing—something that lets no air or water pass through. Clean plastic will work. Tape this dressing down with a corner left free in hopes air collecting under tension in the chest will self-release. If collecting air doesn't release, a **pneumothorax** may develop, and may progress to life-threatening tension. If severe difficulty breathing develops, push your finger, or some object, gently into the hole to release the trapped air. This may all that can save the patient. Once again, a speedy evacuation is critical.

Evacuation Guideline
   Evacuate rapidly anyone with signs and symptoms of serious chest injury and/or anyone with increasing difficulty breathing.

8: Abdominal Injuries

   Abdominal injuries may be generally classified in two categories: 1) **blunt trauma**, a closed abdominal injury caused by a forceful blow to the abdomen, and 2) **penetrating trauma**, an open abdominal injury caused by an object being forced into the abdomen. The extent of injury is often difficult to assess in the backcountry—or anywhere, for that matter. No other region of the human body has more potential to conceal serious blood loss.

Signs and Symptoms of Serious Abdominal Injury

1. Obviously serious abdominal injury, e.g., impaled object, evisceration (internal organs outside the body).
2. Signs and symptoms of shock (*see Shock*).
3. Blood in the vomit, feces, or urine. Blood may appear like "coffee grounds" in the vomit, black and tarry in the feces, reddish in urine.
4. Pain in the abdomen persisting for more than 12 to 24 hours.
5. Localized abdominal pain, especially with guarding, tenderness, rigidity, palpable lumps, distention and/or asymmetry.

Management of Abdominal Injury

As with all patients, treatment should involve maintenance of the airway. Stay alert to the possibility of vomiting. Generally, treat for shock. Patients suffering blunt trauma should be kept in the position of comfort they choose—if no other injuries prevent this—and kept warm. If you are involved in their evacuation, comfort and warmth should be extended to them during the carry. In general, nothing should be given to them by mouth, but on an extended evacuation sips of water, preferably cool, may be necessary to prevent dehydration.

The immediate seriousness of any penetrating abdominal injury, as with blunt trauma, is determined by what got damaged inside and how bad it's bleeding. With severe bleeding, shock is imminent, and immediate evacuation the only chance of salvation. Over time the risk of infection may be high. General treatment of the patient is the same as for a patient suffering blunt abdominal trauma. Specific treatment will vary somewhat depending on the soft tissue involvement. External bleeding should be controlled. Wounds should be cleaned and bandaged. Impaled objects, in almost all cases, should be stabilized in place.

An evisceration, in short-term care, should be covered with sterile dressings soaked in disinfected water to prevent drying out. Check the dressings every two hours to make sure they stay moist. Cover the moist dressings with thick, dry dressings, and rapidly evacuate the patient. In long-term care, over several hours, the exposed intestines will do better if they are flushed clean with disinfected water and "teased" back inside by gently pulling the wound open. If teasing doesn't work, you may have to gently push the exposed loops of intestine back inside the abdominal cavity. Then clean and bandage the wound.

Evacuation Guideline

Evacuate anyone with signs and symptoms of serious abdominal trauma.

9: Wound Management

Note: Before touching blood, or any other body fluid, it is best to put on protective gloves. If there is a chance blood may be splashed into your eyes, wear glasses, e.g., sunglasses.

When you're far from a doctor, three goals will guide
your management of wounds: 1) stop serious bleeding,
2) prevent infection, and 3) promote healing.

Bleeding

Almost all bleeding can be stopped with direct pressure
and elevation: Pressure from your hand directly on the
wound and elevation of the wound above the patient's
heart. If there's time, place a sterile dressing on the wound
before applying pressure. If there's no time, grab anything
absorbent to press into the wound. You can let small
wounds bleed to a stop—which may actually clean them a
bit.

Warning! Some wounds should not be treated with
direct pressure. Pressure to a wound on a patient's neck
may cut off his air supply—stop the bleeding by carefully
pinching the opening closed. Pressure to a head wound may
push cracked bone fragments into his brain—cover the
wound with a bulky dressing and press lightly.

Wound Cleaning

Proper wound cleaning, closing, and dressing almost
equal the prevention of infection. Cleaning also speeds
healing and reduces scarring. Start by washing your own
hands and putting on surgical gloves. Avoid, as much as
possible, breathing into, coughing around, or drooling onto
an open wound.

The best method for cleaning is mechanical irrigation.
Irrigation involves a high pressure stream of an acceptable

solution directed into the wound, best directed from an
irrigation syringe. For most wounds, the best cleaning
solution is plain disinfected water. For heavily
contaminated wounds, you can whip up a disinfecting
solution by thoroughly mixing an ounce of povidone-iodine
in a liter of clean water, and waiting about five minutes.
Note: Don't drink this solution. Draw the solution into the
syringe, hold it two to four inches above the wound and
perpendicular to the wound, and push down forcefully on
the plunger. Keep the wound tipped so the solution runs
out. Use at least half a liter, more if the wound still looks
unclean. Without an irrigation syringe, you can improvise
by using a biking water bottle, melting a pinhole in the
center of the lid of a standard water bottle, or punching a
pinhole in a clean plastic bag. If you use something other
than plain water, follow irrigation with a final flush of
disinfected water.

Wound Closure

After thoroughly cleaning small wounds that gape open,
facial wounds, or scalp wounds, they can be closed with
closure strips or strips of tape. Another guideline is this: If
you had to hold a wound open to thoroughly irrigate it, the
wound should probably be taped shut. If hair gets in the
way, it can be carefully clipped short, but it should not be
shaved. If you have tincture of benzoin compound, smear a
line along both sides of the wound. Benzoin is an irritant so
take care to keep it out of the wound. Let the benzoin dry

for about 30 seconds. Benzoin's stickiness will help keep the closure strips in place. Touch the closure strips only on their ends to avoid contamination. Apply one end of one strip to one side of the wound and another to the opposite side. By using the opposing strips as handles, you can pull the wound edges together, pulling the skin as close as possible to where it should lie naturally.

Note: Large dirty wounds, wound that expose bones, tendons, or ligaments, and wounds caused by animal bites should be left open. They are difficult to clean well enough to prevent infection. After irrigation, cover these wounds with sterile gauze. Exceptionally dirty wounds should be packed open with moist sterile gauze and covered with dry gauze to allow them to drain until a physician can be consulted.

Wound Dressing

The dressing is the primary covering of a wound. It works best if it's sterile, non-adherent, porous, resistant to bacterial invasion, and easy to use. Wounds heal faster with less scarring if they're kept slightly moist with an antibiotic ointment or with a dressing that holds in the body's moisture, such as a micro-thin film dressing. Film dressings have the added advantages of being see-through and water-repelling. The dressing should completely cover the wound and ideally extend a half-inch or so beyond the wound's edge. If you use a micro-thin film dressing, do not use an ointment.

The function of the bandage is to fix, protect, and further assist the dressing. It can be conforming gauze, tape, elastic wraps, clean cotton strips, or improvised out of anything available. The usefulness of a bandage is handicapped if it's too loose, and dangerous if it's too tight. Do not hide rings or anything that could cut off circulation if swelling occurs. Check bandages often.

Notes on Specific Wounds

Bruises (contusions): Usually no problem, but if they're big and over organs watch for signs of internal bleeding (shock). They'll freeze faster than healthy skin in extreme cold.

Lacerations (cuts): Check for imbedded debris. You might have to pick out large contaminants with sterilized tweezers.

Avulsions (flaps): Lift up the flap to irrigate thoroughly underneath. Use closure strips to hold it in place.

Amputations: Save the amputated part, preferably wrapped in moist, sterile gauze, then sealed in a clean plastic bag and placed in ice water.

Impalements: Generally, do not remove them unless they are very loose. Carefully stabilize the object in place.

Abrasions (scrapes): Scrubbing is the best way to clean these shallow dirty wounds. Use of an anesthetic cleansing pad prior to scrubbing can ease the pain a little, but be prepared for a violent reaction in the patient. Irrigate first. Then scrub with a scrub brush or impregnated sponge, e.g., Green Soap Sponge®, or a gauze pad and soap and water.

Irrigate clean. Apply a thin layer of antibiotic ointment. Then a dressing and bandage.

Wound Infection

Check all wounds regularly for signs of infection: 1) increasing pain, heat, redness, and swelling, 2) pus, 3) appearance of red streaks just under the skin near the wound, and 4) systemic fever. If you see signs of infection, open the wound back up, and let it drain. You may need to encourage the process with soaks in water as hot as the patient can tolerate. Pack the wound with moist, sterile gauze to keep it draining, and dress it with dry, sterile gauze. Wet-to-dry dressings encourage draining. Re-clean and re-pack the wound twice a day, if possible. And start looking for a doctor.

Evacuation Guideline

Evacuate anyone with a wound that 1) is heavily contaminated, 2) opens a joint space, 3) involves tendons or ligaments, 4) was caused by an animal bite, 5) is deep and on the face, 6) is deep and affects a special function area such as hands and feet, 7) was caused by a crushing injury, and 8) shows evidence of serious infection.

10: Burns

Burns are among the most painful and emotionally distressing of injuries. Even relatively minor burns may disrupt the wilderness experience of an individual, or an expedition.

Initial Care

1. Remove the patient from the source of the burn.

2. Stop the burning process. The faster the better—within 30 seconds, if possible. Burns can continue to injure tissue for a surprisingly long time. No first aid will be effective until the burning process has stopped. Smother flames, if appropriate, then cool the burn with water. Do not try to remove tar or melted plastic.

3. Manage the ABC's.

4. Assess for associated injuries, e.g., fractures, lacerations.

Evaluate the Burn

Every aspect of burn treatment depends on your assessment of the depth and extent of the injury. Even though this assessment may be rough, it will be your basis for deciding how the patient will be managed, whether evacuation is required, and how urgently.

Depth

BURN ASSESSMENT

Depth	Superficial	Partial Thickness	Full Thickness
Skin Layer	Epidermis	Epidermis/ Dermis	All Layers
Color	Bright Red	Red to pale	Pale (for scalds), charred (for open flame)
Blisters	None	Large, fluid-filled	Dry
Pain	Mild to moderate	Severe	Dull to severe
Healing	Spontaneous 3–5 days	Spontaneous 1–3 weeks	Very slow
Scarring	None	Moderate	Severe

Extent

Use the **Rule of Palmar Surface** (the patient's palmar surface—inner surface of palm and fingers—equals about one percent Total Body Surface Area or TBSA).

Pain

In addition to depth and extent, do not underestimate the value of pain as a burn assessment tool. If the patient is in a lot of pain, that is an indication of the need for a physician's care.

General Treatment for the Burn

1. Gently wash the burn with slightly warm water and mild soap. Pat dry.
2. Remove the skin from blisters that have popped open (but do not open blisters). Wipe away serum and obvious dirt.
3. Dress the burn with a thin layer of antibiotic ointment.
4. Cover the burn with a gauze pad or a thin layer of roll gauze, or apply clean clothing. Covering wounds reduces pain and evaporative losses.

    When evacuation is imminent, do not re-dress or re-examine the injury. But if evacuation is distant, re-dress twice a day by removing old dressings, re-washing (and removing the old ointment), and putting on a clean covering. (**Note:** You may have to soak off old dressings with clean tepid water.)
5. Do not pack wounds or patient in ice.
6. Elevate burned extremities to minimize swelling. Swelling retards healing and encourages infection. Get the patient, as much as possible, to gently and regularly move burned areas immediately, and continue until healing is complete.

7. Ibuprofen is probably the best over-the-counter painkiller for burn pain (including sunburn).
8. If you have no ointment, no dressings, and/or no skill, leave the burn alone. The burn's surface will dry into a scab-like covering that provides a significant amount of protection.

General Treatment for the Patient

1. Keep the patient warm. When skin is lost, so is the patient's ability to thermoregulate.
2. Get the patient to drink as much fluid as they will tolerate, unless drinking makes the patient nauseous. Nausea and vomiting are very common during the first 24 to 48 hours.

Evacuation Guideline

Evacuate all patients with serious burns to the face, neck, hands, feet, armpits or groin, and all patients with full thickness burns. Rapidly evacuate all patients with burns threatening the airway, with circumferential burns, and with blisters and/or full thickness burns covering 15 percent TBSA.

11: Musculoskeletal Injuries
Strains

Strains are overstretched muscles and/or the tendons that attach muscles to bones. They can range from a mild annoyance to debilitating. A strain can be used within the limits of pain—in other words, if it hurts, don't do it. RICE can be helpful (*see below Sprains*).

If **lower back pain** came on suddenly, apply cold for 20 to 30 minutes, several times a day, for the first 48 hours. If the pain grew gradually, heat usually works best. After two days, heat is best in most cases. Patient should rest on his or her side, or on the back with high padding beneath the knees. The patient will heal faster by taking a non-steroidal anti-inflammatory drug, e.g., ibuprofen. Massages help. Reasons to evacuate a back-strained patient include: 1) the pain (or numbness) begins to radiate all the way down an arm or leg, 2) the pain remains strong even when the injured area is at rest, 3) the pain started as a result of illness, and 4) the pain came on sharply after a fall from a height or a sudden jolting stop.

Sprains

Sprains are injuries to ligaments, the bands holding bones to bones at joints, and can vary from simple overstretching to complete tears. Unlike fractures that mend strong, and strains that heal well, a sprain may come back to haunt you the rest of your life, especially if you treat it improperly. What's really unfortunate about sprains is that they don't hurt as much as they should. Pain would encourage sensible action. Sensible action has three stages: First Aid, Rest, and Retraining.

Note: Strains and sprains, especially where a joint is involved, are virtually impossible to differentiate. Differentiation, however, is not required. They are both treated the same.

First aid is **RICE**: **R**est, **I**ce, **C**ompression and **E**levation. But RICE should be applied after an initial evaluation of the injury. The primary goal of the evaluation is to determine if the injury is usable or not. Get the patient at rest and relaxed—and take a look at the injury. Look for deformities and rapid swelling and discoloration. Have the patient actively move the joint and evaluate the amount of pain involved. Move the joint more aggressively with your hands and evaluate the pain response. Finally, if the joint appears useable, have the patient test it with his or her body weight. A useable injury can be, well, used. An un-useable injury will require a splint *(see below)*.

Useable or un-useable, stay off the injury (Rest) for the first half hour while you reduce its temperature (Ice) as much as possible without freezing. Crushed ice works best. It conforms to the shape of the anatomy involved. Do **not** put ice directly on skin—put it in a plastic bag and wrap it in a shirt or sock. Without ice, soak in cold water, or carry chemical cold packs, or (during warmer months) wrap the joint in wet cotton and let evaporation cool the damaged area. Compression (C) requires an elastic wrap. Wrap it

snug but not tight enough to cut off healthy circulation.
Elevation (E) refers to keeping the injury higher than the
patient's heart. After 20 to 30 minutes of RICE, remove the
treatment and let the joint warm naturally for 10 to 15
minutes before use. (Note: The injury will heal faster if
RICE is repeated three or four times a day until pain and
swelling subside.)

The patient will benefit also from adequate hydration
and regular use of an anti-inflammatory drug such as
ibuprofen. After RICE, a splint that allows the joint to
function will aid the patient.

A walking-splint for the knee should hold the knee in
place without putting pressure on the kneecap. A pad
should be placed behind the knee within the splint to keep
the knee slightly flexed.

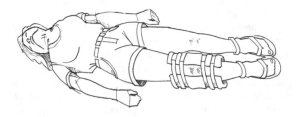

Figure 9: Walking Splint for Knee

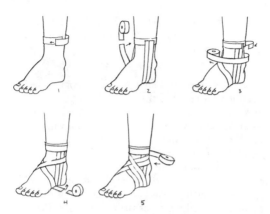

Figure 10: Ankle Taping

Ankle taping should be applied firmly but not tight enough to cut off circulation. Tape should be applied as 1) "stirrups" to pull the bones of the ankle together bottom to top, and 2) "figure of eights" to pull the bones of the ankle together side to side.

Even mild sprains may take a long time to heal completely—but the injury might feel comfortable in a week or less. Exercise sprains when they start to feel okay, but do **not** push past the point of pain. How do you know when you're well? Starting with gentle exercise and working up, compare the injured side to the uninjured side. Is the balance the same? The strength the same? Is the pain

51

tolerance the same? When you are bilaterally equal for approximately 10 repetitions of the same movement, you are usually ready to aggressively retrain.

Fractures

Broken bones make up a large percentage of injuries in the backcountry. Sometimes the assessment is simple: Bones stick out through the skin, joints are created where no joint should exist. Without the obvious, and without an x-ray, rescuers can base an assessment on common sense and a good **LAF** at the patient.

L stands for **Look**. Remove or cut away clothing carefully, and take a look at the site of the injury. (In cold weather, reduce "cutting away" to a minimum.) Is there discoloration and swelling? Does the patient move the injury easily or guard it jealously? Compare the injured side to the uninjured side. Does it **look** broken?

A stands for **Ask**. Ask the patient: How did the injury occur? (High speed impacts cause more damage that low speed impacts.) Do you think you're broken? (The patient is often right.) How bad does it hurt? (Surrounding muscle spasms create pain and give evidence of the seriousness of the injury.)

F stands for **Feel**. Gently touch the damaged area. Does the patient react to your touch? (Ouch!) Does it feel like the muscles are spasming? Does it feel unstable? Is there "point tenderness"—one particular spot that hurts noticeably more when touched? These are indications of a fracture.

Check for **C**irculation, **S**ensation and **M**otion (CSM) beyond the site of the injury. Loss of a pulse, numbness, tingling, and inability to move are signs of loss of normal blood flow and loss of normal nerve messages—serious complications with a fracture. After splinting, check CSM often to assure circulation is not cut off by wraps that are too tight.

Splinting

The general rule is: **When in doubt, splint!** A splint should immobilize the broken bone(s), prevent further injury, and maximize patient comfort until a medical facility can be reached. To do this best, a splint needs to be made of 1) something to pad the injury comfortably, and 2) something rigid enough to provide support. Padding should fill all the spaces within the system to prevent movement of the injury. **Avoid the Void!** In addition, a splint should be long enough to 3) immobilize the joints above and below a broken bone, or immobilize the bones above and below an injured joint.

Splints should immobilize the injury in the position of function, or as close to position of function as possible. Functional positions include: 1) spine, including neck and pelvis, straight with padding in the small of the back, 2) legs almost straight with padding behind the knees for slight flexion, 3) feet at 90° to legs, 4) arms flexed at 90°, and 5) hands in a functional curve with padding in the palms.

In choosing materials for splinting, you are only limited by imagination: sleeping bags, foamlite pads (and they can be cut to fit the problem), extra clothing, soft debris from the forest floor stuffed into extra clothing. For rigidity there are items such as sticks, tent poles, ski poles, ice axes, Crazy Creek Chairs®, internal and external pack frames. Lightweight commercial splints are available as additions to your first aid kit (e.g., SAM Splint®, wire splints). Splints can be secured in place with things like bandannas, strips of clothing, pack straps, belts, and rope. Useful items in your first aid kit for securing splints include tape, elastic wraps, and roll gauze. Large triangular bandages are helpful in creating slings and swathes.

Specific Fractures

Jaw Fractures can be held in place with a wide wrap that goes around the head. Be sure the wrap can be removed quickly if the patient feels like vomiting.

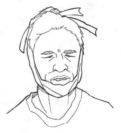

Figure 11: Jaw Splint

Collar-bone Fractures can be secured with a sling-and-swathe. Slings can be made from triangular bandages, or improvised by lifting the tail of the patient's shirt up over the

arm on the injured side and safety-pinning it in place. Be
sure the sling lifts the elbow to take pressure off the
shoulder.

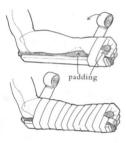

Lower Arm Fractures
(including wrist and hand) can
be secured to a well-padded rigid
support, then held in a sling-
and-swathe. Place a roll of
something soft in the hand to
keep it in position of function. If
bones of the hand are damaged,
be sure to secure the hand well
to the splint with, as always, lots
of padding.

Figure 12: Arm Splint

Fingers that are broken can be secured to nearby
healthy fingers with padding between the fingers.

Upper Arm Fractures can be placed in a sling-and-
swathe. Leaving the elbow free sometimes eases the pain.
Secure the broken bone to the patient's chest wall with a
wide soft wrap.

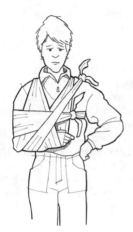
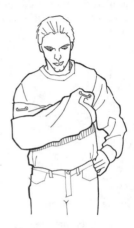

Figure 13: Sling and Swathe   *Figure 14: Shirt as Sling*

Rib Fractures can be protected by supporting the arm on the injured side with a sling-and-swathe. Do **not** wrap a band snugly around the patient's chest. **Do** encourage the patient regularly to take deep breaths, even if it hurts, to keep the lungs clear. Be sure to watch the patient for increasing difficulty breathing *(see Chest Injuries)*.

Pelvis and Hip Fractures should include securing the entire patient on a rigid litter before attempting a carry-out. Conforming wraps around the pelvis may provide some comfort. Secure the legs comfortably to each other. Be sure to watch the patient for signs of shock due to internal bleeding common with pelvic fractures.

Lower Leg Fractures (including the ankle and foot) can be secured on a well-padded rigid support that includes immobilization of the ankle and foot. Foamlite sleeping pads and Crazy Creek Chairs® make excellent lower leg splints. Pad behind the knee for comfort.

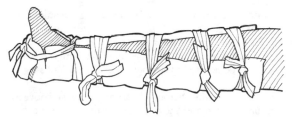

Figure 15: Lower Leg Splint

Thigh (Femur) Fractures should get gentle traction-in-line as soon as possible. Prompt manual traction is required to 1) prevent further injury from movement or massive spasms of the large thigh muscles, 2) reduce bleeding into the thigh, which can be severe even without an open wound, and 3) reduce pain, which can be extreme. **Maintain manual traction until a traction splint is in place.** Splinting a fractured femur requires a device that maintains traction on the leg. Commercial products are available (such as the Kendrick Traction Device®—KTD for short), but such a device can be improvised in the field. Several methods of improvising traction exist.

Here's one:

1. One rescuer should hold traction **at all times** while a second rescuer gathers material.
2. Create a fixation splint beneath or around the patient's thigh.
3. A hitch or harness needs to be created at the ankle on the injured side.
4. A shaft (stick, ski pole, paddle, tent pole, etc.) approximately 18 inches longer than the patient's leg needs to be secured to the outside of the patient's leg at hip level.
5. With rope, cord, or strong cloth apply traction between the ankle hitch and the outer end of the shaft via a trucker's hitch until the mechanical traction is equal to or greater than the manual traction. (The patient is a good judge of the amount of traction.)
6. Secure the system, backing up knots, padding all possible pressure points.
7. An evacuation via a rigid litter, as soon as possible, is required.

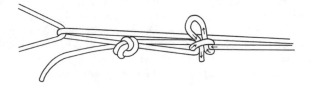

Figure 16: Trucker's Hitch

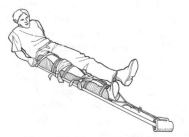

Figure 17: Traction Splint

Complicated Fractures

An **Angulated Fracture** (angles in bones in the wrong place) needs to be realigned to normal anatomical position. Pull gentle traction on the broken bone **along the line in which it lies.** This relaxes the muscles and reduces the pain allowing you to move the broken bone slowly and gently back into normal alignment. The sooner this movement takes place the better. Do **not** use force. Do **not** continue if the patient complains of increasing pain. Once aligned, splint as usual. If alignment cannot be achieved, splint as best you can.

An **Open Fracture** is indicated by an open wound over the fracture. Bones may or may not be visible. All open fractures should be seen by a physician as soon as possible. The wound should be irrigated and dressed appropriately (*see Wound Management*), and the bone should be splinted. If bone ends stick out of the wound, and if the doctor is far away: 1) clean the wound and bone ends without scrubbing, 2) apply gentle traction-in-line to the fracture and pull the bone ends back under the skin, 3) dress the wound, and 4) splint. Infection is on the way, but bones live longer inside the body.

Dislocations

With a dislocation, the bone ends in a joint are no longer properly aligned. The patient typically experiences pain in the joint, and a loss of normal range of motion. The joint looks "wrong." If a doctor is nearby, splint the joint in order to stabilize it in the position found. When the doctor is far away, attempt to reduce (relocate) the dislocation before splinting.

Work quickly but calmly. Typically, the sooner a reduction is attempted, the easier it is on patient and rescuer. Encourage the patient to relax as much as possible, with special concentration on relaxing the injured joint. Place yourself in a position that will allow you to pull gentle traction-in-line. With a firm grip on both sides of the dislocated joint (sometimes two rescuers are required), pull **along the lines in which the bones lie**. Under gentle traction, move the bones toward normal alignment. **Do not use force. Stop if pain increases.** Once reduced, the injury should be splinted *(see above)*.

Specific Dislocations

Jaw Dislocations can be reduced by wrapping something soft around your thumbs, e.g., gauze, reaching into the patient's mouth, and pressing down and forward with your thumbs on the back molars.

Cervical Spine (Neck) Dislocations qualify as a possible spinal cord injury, and should be treated as such (*see Spine Injuries*).

Shoulder Dislocations are one of the most common. There are several ways to reduce a dislocated shoulder.

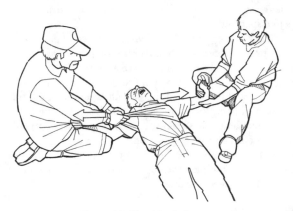

Figure 18: Shoulder Relocation

Here is a proven-safe one:
1. With the patient lying on the ground, have a second rescuer sit opposite the damaged shoulder and hold counter-traction via the patient's clothing or by

wrapping something, e.g., a long-sleeved shirt, around the patient's chest to hold on to.

2. The first rescuer pulls gentle traction-in-line on the arm on the injured side, keeping the patient's elbow flexed.

3. Under traction, move the arm up and out, mimicking the motion the arm would go through if a baseball was being thrown, until the arm is at 90° to the patient's body.

4. Hold traction until the shoulder reduces. Gently rotating the arm at the shoulder may aid reduction.

5. Sling-and-swathe the arm.

Here is another one, but you might have a long wait for reduction:

1. Have the patient prone (face down) across a rock or log with the arm on the injured side dangling down vertically.

2. With a soft cloth, tie something of about 15 pounds weight to the dangling wrist.

3. Wait.

Wrist Dislocations are usually associated with a fracture of the wrist. Reduction is typically simple. Splint well.

Finger Dislocations are also common. Keeping the injured finger partially flexed, pull on the end while pressing the dislocated joint back into place with your other thumb. Tape the injured finger to a neighbor with a gauze pad between them. Do **not** tape directly over the joint itself.

Knee Dislocations usually leave the knee useless for walking. With gentle traction, move the leg to normal alignment, splint securely, and figure out how to carry the patient.

Patella (Kneecap) Dislocations are typically very easy to reduce. Apply gentle traction to the leg to straighten it out. Sometimes the kneecap pops back into place when the leg is straightened. If it doesn't, massage the thigh and push the kneecap gently back into normal alignment with your hand. With a splint that does not put pressure on the kneecap, the patient can usually walk out.

Ankle Dislocations will usually involve fractured bones and easy reduction. Reduction can usually be achieved by taking hold of the patient's toes and lifting until the weight of the leg acts as counter-traction. A gentle pull on the heel may be required. Splint well.

Toe Dislocations are treated the same as fingers.

Other joints, of course, may be dislocated. More advanced training should be acquired before attempting more complex reductions. Monitor all dislocations after splinting. Most patients should see a physician as soon as possible. Exceptions might include fingers and toes, patellas, and chronic dislocations that the patient is able to use with reasonable comfort after the reduction.

Evacuation Guideline

With a useable injury, the degree of discomfort of the patient will determine more than anything the need to evacuate the patient. Evacuate all patients with un-useable injuries, with first-time dislocations, and with injuries that create a decrease in circulation beyond the injury.

12: Hypothermia

Since hypothermia, low heat in the body's core, subtly steals your ability to make a rational decision, it is probably related to more backcountry injuries and deaths than any other cause.

Signs of Hypothermia

1. **Gross coordination is lost**, and patient begins to stumble.

2. **A brain dulled by the cold**, and patient drops gear and doesn't notice, loses direction and doesn't care, feels cold but does nothing about it. Difficult to detect in others, this is very difficult to detect in yourself.

3. **Loss of control of fine motor skills**, and patient can't buckle buckles, zip up her or his parka, strike a match to start a stove. The brain is trying to save itself by shunting blood away from less important body parts such as hands and feet.

4. **Uncontrollable shivering** starts when the core reaches approximately 95° F. Shivering produces heat, but it requires a high energy output to maintain. If the heat isn't trapped near the body, or energy replenished with food, or both, core temperature continues to drop ever faster.

5. **Shivering stops,** and patient enters what may be termed a "metabolic icebox": The body grows progressively more rigid, colder and colder to touch, with slowing and weakening pulse and respirations that may become impossible to detect. Although a person can survive for hours, perhaps days, in this deteriorating condition, the eventual end is death unless quality care is provided.

Management of Hypothermia

Management can be divided, for simplicity, into two categories: 1) treatment for mild hypothermia, and 2) treatment for severe hypothermia.

The **mild hypothermia** patient is still trying to warm up internally. The patient can talk, eat, and shiver. Change the environment so the heat being produced internally is not lost. Get the patient out of wet clothes and into something dry, out of wind and cold and into some kind of shelter, even if the only shelter available in the protection of waterproof, windproof clothing. Cover the patient's head and neck where critical heat is easily lost. If the patient can take food and drink, and eat and drink, give her or him simple carbohydrates to stoke the inner fire. Fluids are more important than solids to a cold person. A warm (not hot) sweet drink will add a tiny bit of heat and a lot of simple sugar for energy. Even cold fluids are better than no fluids. If the patient can still exercise easily, keep moving after initial treatment. If the patient can't exercise easily, do all you can to encourage entrapment of inner heat production: insulate the patient from the ground, bundle in dry insulation, snuggle with warm people, place hot water bottles in the hands or at the feet (but not against naked skin), use chemical heat packs as you would hot water bottles—and wait until the patient returns to normal.

The **severe hypothermia** patient is semi-conscious or unconscious, and has stopped shivering. She or he has lost the ability to rewarm. Handle the patient gently—roughness can overload a cold heart, and stop it. Remove clothing and bundle the patient up in as much dry insulation as possible. Insulate well from the ground. Wrap hot water bottles or heat packs in dry socks or shirts and place them appropriately: palms of hands, soles of feet, armpits, groin—in that order. Finish with a vapor barrier—a tent fly, sheet of plastic, garbage bags—something to trap any heat still left in the patient. The final product is a cocoon, a "hypothermia wrap" open only to the mouth and nose. Do **not** try to force food or drink. Treat for severe hypothermia even if the patient appears dead. **No patient is dead, as far as you're concerned, unless he or she is warm and dead.** If the patient appears dead, perform artificial respirations for 5–15 minutes before any movement of the patient. Wrap them as described above—and go for help.

Prevention of Hypothermia

1. Wear clothing that retains body heat even when wet.
2. Stay dry by wearing layers of clothing, taking off layers before sweating starts, adding them back before chilling occurs.
3. Drink lots of water.
4. Eat lots, especially carbohydrates.
5. Maintain a pace that prevents overexertion. Rest often.
6. In a group, watch each other for signs of hypothermia. Treat early, and if one person is treated, treat everyone.

Evacuation Guideline

Evacuate with extreme gentleness anyone with severe hypothermia.

13: Frostbite

Frostbite is localized freezing of tissue, and it often walks frigid hand-in-hand with hypothermia. Proper treatment of frostbite can save near-frozen tissue and reduce the extent of already-frozen tissue.

Partial-Thickness Frostbite

Skin is pale and numb, but it moves when you press on it. Passive warming should begin immediately. In the field, cover the cold body part with warm body parts. Cover your nose with your warm hand, stick your cold hand against your warm stomach, put your cold toes against the warm stomach of a friend. Do **not** rub the cold skin. Do **not** place cold skin near a hot heat source because numb tissue is very susceptible to heat injury. Give ibuprofen, if available, and lots of water to drink.

Skin that looks OK after rewarming is usually OK. If blisters form after warming, a physician should be consulted as soon as possible. In the meantime, two things should be remembered: 1) Leave the bubble intact. It protects the underlying tissue, and creates less of a chance for infection. 2) Blisters re-freeze quickly, multiplying the damage. Be careful to prevent re-freezing.

Full-Thickness Frostbite

Skin is pale and numb, and hard. Normal field conditions make warming of deep frostbite impractical. The most reasonable treatment is to remove all clothing, e.g., socks, mittens, unless it's frozen to the skin. Gently bundle the frozen skin in lots of dry insulation—and evacuate the patient.

If re-freezing is unlikely, and you have the means available, full-thickness frostbite is best treated by rapid warming in water of approximately 104° to 108°F (40° to 42°C). Too hot and heat damage occurs. Too cold and rewarming is too slow for maximum benefit. Warming is usually accomplished in 30 to 40 minutes, but it's better to err on the side of caution and rewarm longer than necessary rather than less than necessary. Soft cotton should be placed between thawed digits, but, otherwise, contact with anything should be avoided. Pain is often intense, and painkillers should be started prior to thawing. Ibuprofen started as soon as possible seems to reduce the extent of damage to tissue. Keep the patient well-hydrated. Prevention of re-freezing is of paramount importance. Find a doctor as soon as possible.

Prevention of Frostbite

Follow the same guidelines that prevent hypothermia. Avoid snug clothing that restricts circulation, especially on the feet and hands. Wear clothing appropriate for cold weather, e.g., insulated boots, mittens rather than gloves. Be careful to protect your skin from wind and contact with cold metal and cold gasoline. Avoid alcohol and tobacco. If your toes hurt from the cold, rejoice, and stop and rewarm them before they go numb with the possibility of permanent injury.

Evacuation Guideline

Evacuate patients with blisters and/or full-thickness frostbite.

14: Heat Illness

Heat illness describes a wide range of problems associated with a rise in air temperature—everything from feeling hot and tired to the life-threat of heat stroke. In addition to rising temperatures, other factors increase your risk of heat illness: 1) high humidity, 2) being overweight, 3) being very young or very old, 4) being unaccustomed to

heat, 5) taking certain drugs, such as antihistamines
(consult your physician), and, 6) the most important factor,
being dehydrated.

Heat Exhaustion

The patient has been exercising, and sweating out
water and salt, and he or she feels very tired. Skin may
appear pale and sweaty, and the patient complains of a
headache, perhaps nausea and sometimes vomiting.
Dizziness may strike when the patient stands quickly. An
elevated heart rate is common. Overall, the patient may
feel like he or she had a sudden attack of the flu.

The problem is a volume problem—not enough water
inside the patient—and it's typically not serious. Core
temperature may have risen a few degrees, or none at all.
The cure is suggested by the name of the condition:
Exhaustion calls for rest, preferably in a cool, shady spot.
Replace lost fluids with water, and lost salt by adding a
pinch to a liter of water or munching salty snacks. Use of
oral rehydration salts may speed recovery. Do **not** use salt
tablets—they are too concentrated. To increase the rate of
cooling, the patient may be wet down and fanned. A
drowsy patient may be allowed to sleep. When the patient
feels OK, he or she may continue the backcountry
adventure.

Heat Cramps

Associated with heat exhaustion are heat cramps, most
commonly occurring in the large muscles of the legs, and

71

sometimes extending up into the abdomen. Though the discomfort may be great, the problem is rarely serious. Treatment includes rest, gentle stretching and massage, and drinking water, preferably with a pinch of salt added per liter or with a salty snack. Once again, oral rehydration salts may speed recovery. Once feeling well, the patient may continue. But if the cramps return, the sufferer should take the rest of the day off. Overworking depleted muscles can lead to permanent injury.

Heat Stroke

Pushing past a minor heat illness can lead to the major problem of heat stroke. The patient's inability to shed heat faster than gaining it produces a rise in core temperature to 105°F (40.5°C) or more. Disorientation and bizarre personality changes are common signs. Skin turns hot and red and sometimes (but far from always) dry. Look for a fast heart rate, fast breathing, and complaints of a headache.

Heat stroke is a temperature problem. The patient is too hot inside. Once a human brain gets that hot, it is a **true emergency**, and only rapid cooling will save the patient. Take off any heat-retaining clothes and drench the patient with water. Concentrate cooling efforts on the head and neck. Cold packs may be used on the palms of the hands, the soles of the feet, the head, neck, armpits, groin. Fan the patient constantly to increase evaporation. Massage the limbs to encourage cooler blood to return to the core. When, or if, the patient is able to accept and drink cold water, give it. Do **not** give fever-reducing drugs.

The patient must see a doctor as soon as possible, even if she or he appears to have recovered. During evacuation, a careful watch on the patient should be maintained. Relapses are common.

Hyponatremia

You can drink too much water—if you're not eating. Salt loss in sweat exceeding salt intake plus water intake exceeding water loss equals lowered sodium level in the blood. When blood sodium gets too low, you have a case of hyponatremia.

Common complaints include headache, weakness, fatigue, lightheadedness, muscle cramps, nausea with or without vomiting, sweaty skin, normal core temperature, normal or slightly elevated pulse and respirations, and a bit of anxiety. Sound familiar? Yep, it sounds like heat exhaustion. But if you treat it like heat exhaustion—just add water—you are harming the hyponatremia patient. More severe symptoms of hyponatremia include a patient who is disoriented, irritable, and combative—which gives the problem a more common name: water intoxication. Untreated, the ultimate result will be seizures, coma, and death.

Heat exhausted patients typically have a low output of yellowish urine (urinating every 6-8 hours) combined with thirst. Hyponatremia patients have urinated recently and the urine was probably clear. Hyponatremia patients will also claim to have been drinking a lot of water, and they deny thirst.

Patients with mild to moderate symptoms and a normal mental status may be treated in the field: Rest in shade with no fluid intake and a gradual intake of salty foods while the kidneys reestablish a sodium balance. Once a patient develops hunger and thirst combined with normal urine output, the problem is solved. Restriction of fluids for someone who is well hydrated, fortunately, is harmless. Concerning patients with an altered mental status there is no question: They demand rapid evacuation to a medical facility.

Prevention of Heat Illness

1. Stay well-hydrated. Urine output should be clear and relatively copious, an indication of adequate hydration. Water or diluted sports drinks are best to drink. It is practically impossible to drink too much water (see above Hyponatremia). Avoid alcohol and caffeinated drinks.
2. Munch on lightly salted snacks.
3. Wear baggy, loosely-woven clothing that allows evaporation of sweat. Keep your head covered.
4. Keep yourself fit, and allow time for acclimatization when you're new to a hot environment. Go slow the first few days and avoid the hottest times of day.
5. Beware drugs that increase your risk of heat illness.
6. Rest often in the shade.

Evacuation Guideline

Evacuate anyone who has an altered mental status due to heat or hyponatremia.

15: Lightning Injuries

The danger of the awesome and unpredictable power of lightning cannot be overemphasized. To maximize your safety, follow these guidelines:

1. **Know local weather patterns.** Lightning storms, in general, tend to roll in quickly in the afternoon of summer months.

2. **Plot storms.** When the flash of lightning precedes the boom of thunder by five seconds, the storm is approximately one mile away, and you should already have found a safe spot to wait out the storm.

3. **Find a safe spot.** Avoid high places, high objects, metal objects, open places, low places, and open bodies of water. Seek uniform cover, e.g., low rolling hills or trees of about the same size, deep dry caves, buildings, cars with the windows rolled up.

4. **Assume a safe position when outdoors.** Squat or sit in a tight position

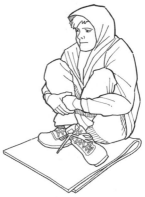

Figure 19:
Lightning Protection Position

on insulating material. Spread groups out, but try to keep everyone in sight.

A lightning strike may produce several types of patients: 1) the thoroughly and obviously dead, 2) non-breathing patients who respond well to rescue breathing, 3) pulseless, non-breathing patients who may respond to CPR, 4) the battered around who have sustained treatable injuries, and 5) the stunned who are not really hurt at all. After a lightning strike, assess and treat first those patients who appear dead—they might be recoverable.

Evacuation Guideline
Evacuate all patients who have been struck by lightning, even if they appear to be OK soon after the injury. Serious problems sometimes develop later.

16: Drowning

No situation has more inherent danger for rescuers than one in which someone is drowning. Follow these guidelines for getting the drowning person safely out of the water:

1. **Reach** with your hand or foot, clothing, a stick, paddle, or anything that allows you to remain safely on land or in a boat.
2. **Throw** something to the person that floats.
3. **Row** to the person, or access the person in some sort of watercraft.
4. **Tow** the person to safety by throwing a line out and hauling him or her in.

5. **Go** if all else fails, and if you've been trained in swimming rescues, but go knowing you risk your life.

Once the patient is safely out of the water, check for breathing. If necessary, begin rescue breathing. There is no value in attempting to clear the patient's lungs of water, but be ready to roll him or her to clear the airway if water or vomit comes up. Check for signs of a beating heart, and begin CPR if necessary. All patients surviving a near-drowning incident should be warmed and evacuated as soon as possible, even if they appear fully recovered. Long-term problems often develop.

In **cold water near-drownings**, patients have been resuscitated after over an hour of submersion, their spark of life kept alive, probably, by the rapid onset of hypothermia. If possible, keep CPR going on cold water submersion patients until help arrives.

Evacuation Guideline

Evacuate anyone who was unconscious, no matter how short a time, during a submersion incident.

17. Bites and Stings
Small Insects

The little biters (mosquitoes, black flies, gnats, etc.) are the most bother but the least serious (except in countries where mosquitoes are still a primary source of disease). Bites can be prevented by wearing: 1) Clothing they can't bite through (**Note:** Darker colors appear to offer some repellent qualities). 2) Insect repellents on skin. Follow the directions on the label carefully with all products, especially with products containing DEET. 3) Permethrin products on clothing. And 4) mud. A wipe with a sting relief pad can ease the itching. Antihistamines, especially diphenhydramine (sold often as Benadryl®) can reduce itching and swelling of more severe reactions.

Bees and Their Relatives

The stinger left by honeybees should be removed as soon as possible. Any means to get it out is acceptable. Immediate use of a Sawyer Extractor® will remove some of the venom but not the stinger. Ice or cold packs on the site of stings from bees, wasps, yellow jackets, hornets, and fire ants will relieve pain and reduce swelling. Diphenhydramine may be given for itching and swelling. Watch the patient for an allergic reaction (see *Medical Emergencies, Allergic Reactions*) to bees and their relatives.

Spiders

Shiny with an hourglass-shape almost always on the abdomen, **black widows** have a bite that often goes unnoticed, but local pain and redness show up at the bite site within an hour. Pain from muscle cramping usually develops in the arm or leg bitten and in the abdomen and back. The pain may be incredibly severe. Fever, chills, sweating and nausea may develop. Ice or cold packs applied to the bite site usually provide some relief. Painkilling drugs may be used, if available. Although most patients recover within 24 hours, evacuation to a doctor is strongly recommended, especially for children and the elderly.

Recluse (fiddleback) spiders have a violin-shape on their back and a bite that usually produces local pain and blister formation within a few hours. A "bulls-eye" of discoloration often surrounds the blister. The blister ruptures, eventually, leaving a growing ulcer of skin destruction. Ice or cold packs can relieve local pain. Painkilling drugs may be useful. If the blister ruptures, treat the open wound appropriately (*see Wound Management*). The patient should be seen by a physician for consideration of drug treatment to minimize damage.

Scorpions

Scorpion stings produce immediate pain and swelling. Sometimes the patient will develop numbness around the sting site. Ice or cold packs will reduce pain. Diphenhydramine can be given for swelling and itching. The patient will soon recover—except sometimes from the sting of *Centruroides*, a southwestern scorpion that may produce a systemic reaction characterized by unusual anxiety, sweating, salivation, gastrointestinal distress, and, most importantly, respiratory distress. No specific first aid is useful for *Centruroides* stings, and immediate evacuation should take place.

Ticks

Ticks may carry diseases that they can pass to humans. Insect repellents repel ticks, and ticks crawling around on your skin do not transmit diseases until they dig in and feed for hours to days. Careful "tick checks" (which can be fun in some groups) should be performed at least twice a day in tick-infected country, and early removal of imbedded ticks prevents the transmission of many diseases. They should be removed gently with tweezers, without excess squeezing, by taking hold of the tick as near the skin as possible and pulling straight out. Any other removal method increases the risk of germ transmission. If a little of the patient's "skin" comes off with the tick, you have done well. If possible, save the tick for evaluation in case of illness in the patient. Wash the little wound. A swipe with an antiseptic may be useful. Watch the patient carefully for signs and symptoms of illness, e.g., rash, fever, which should send the patient to a doctor immediately.

Snakes

A **pit viper** (rattlesnake, water moccasin, or copperhead) bites with either or both retractable fangs producing immediate local pain and swelling within approximately 15 minutes. Blister formation and discoloration usually occur, and may lead to local skin destruction. Patients often report lip-tingling and a funny taste in their mouth within an hour or so. Muscle twitching may result. Death is rare.

Coral snakes (bright red-on-yellow may kill fellow…or a woman) have to gnaw a few moments to deposit venom from non-retractable fixed fangs. Burning pain at the bite site is often followed by pain, tingling, or numbness extending up from the bite—but these signs and symptoms make take up to 12 hours to develop. Serious systemic manifestations include difficulty speaking, swallowing, seeing and breathing. Bites are far less common, and far more dangerous.

After a Snakebite
1. Get away from the snake.
2. Remain as calm as possible.
3. Remove anything might restrict circulation when swelling occurs, e.g., rings.
4. If you have a Sawyer Extractor®, use it as soon as possible. Rapid use may remove a significant amount of venom.
5. Gently wash the bite site.
6. Splint the bitten arm or leg, and keep the bite site on a level with the patient's heart.
7. Transport the patient to a doctor.
8. Do **not** use cold packs, tourniquets, cutting-and-sucking, or electrical shocks.

Rabies

The rabies virus is ultimately lethal once it reaches the brain. Highly suspect animals include bats, raccoons, foxes, skunks, the canines, the felines, and any mammal acting unnaturally. Reduce the risk of any infection from any animal bite by immediate and aggressive wound cleaning and keeping the wound open to allow draining. In a suspect animal bite, seek medical attention as soon as possible for preventive drug therapy.

18: Altitude Illness

When you go higher in altitude, the amount of oxygen available in each breath grows lower. If you go too high too fast, problems may occur. For simplicity, these problems can be divided into two categories: mild and severe.

Mild Altitude Illness

Anyone coming from lower altitudes to 8000 feet or more may complain of headache, unusual fatigue, nausea, loss of appetite, difficulty sleeping, unusual shortness of breath when exercising, and lassitude. The best treatment is: **Do not go up until the symptoms go down.** Exercise lightly and drink plenty of water. Acetazolamide may be used for treatment after symptoms appear. **Consult your physician.** Do **not** use acetazolamide if you're allergic to sulfa drugs. If the symptoms do not go down within two days, the patient should.

Severe Altitude Illness

Untreated, mild illness may progress to severe. The most important early sign of this progression is ataxia (loss of coordination). An ataxic patient cannot walk a straight line or stand straight with feet together and eyes closed. Severe altitude illness may show up as High Altitude Pulmonary Edema (HAPE): constant shortness of breath, chest pain, productive cough, very fast heart rate. Or it may show up as High Altitude Cerebral Edema (HACE): severe headache unrelieved by rest and medication, bizarre changes in personality, perhaps coma. Or it may show up as both. The patient needs to **Go Down**. In addition to descent, the best treatment is supplemental oxygen. Treatment may also include: 1) The drug nifedipine (sold often as Procardia®) for HAPE. 2) The drug dexamethasone (sold often as Decadron®) for HACE. **Consult your physician.** If descent is delayed, use of the Gamow Bag®, a portable hyperbaric chamber that simulates descent, may save the patient's life. Do **not** use a Gamow Bag® instead of descent.

Prevention of Altitude Illness

1. Above 8000–10,000 feet ascend no faster than your ability to acclimatize—an average of 1000 feet per 24 hours of sleeping gain (sleep no more than 1000 feet higher than the night before).

2. Drink plenty of water.
3. Exercise lightly every day.
4. Eat plenty of carbohydrate-rich low-fat foods.
5. Consult your physician about the uses of acetazolamide to prevent mild illness, nifedipine to prevent HAPE, and dexamethasone to prevent mild illness and HACE.

Evacuation Guideline

Rapid descent and/or evacuation is recommended for all patients with signs and symptoms of severe altitude illness.

19: Medical Emergencies
Abdominal Pain

Anything from freeze-dried food to a raging appendicitis can cause complaints of abdominal pain. You may never know the source of the problem. For that reason, it is recommended to evacuate any patient with abdominal pain if:

1. The pain is associated with the signs and symptoms of shock (*see Shock*).
2. The pain persists for longer than 12 to 24 hours.
3. The pain localizes, and especially if the pain involves guarding (the patient voluntarily or involuntarily protects the area), tenderness, abdominal rigidity and/or distention.

4. Blood appears in the vomit, feces, or urine. In vomit it will look like coffee grounds, in the stool black like tar, in the urine a reddish color.
5. Nausea, vomiting, and/or diarrhea persist for longer than 24 to 72 hours.
6. The pain is associated with a fever above 102°F (39°C).
7. The pain is associated with pregnancy.
8. The patient is unable to eat or drink, unable to stay well hydrated.

If you decide the patient's condition is serious, evacuation should be gentle, with the patient in a position of greatest comfort, avoiding anything my mouth except small sips of cold water if the evacuation will be long.

Allergic Reactions

Almost anything eaten, injected into, absorbed by, or breathed in by a person can cause an allergic reaction. For simplicity, allergic reactions can be divided into two stages: mild and severe. Mild reactions are characterized by stuffy noses, itching, swelling and/or hives. They can be treated in the field with an antihistamine, diphenhydramine (sold often as Benadryl®) being a well-accepted choice.

A severe reaction, known as **anaphylaxis**, is a **true emergency**. Anaphylaxis may produce shock but is more typified by extreme difficulty breathing. The patient's only salvation lies in an immediate injection of epinephrine (adrenaline). Injectable epinephrine is available commercially in spring-loaded syringes that function when pressed into the thigh and manually-operated syringes. Everyone who knows they are susceptible to severe allergic reactions should carry injectable epinephrine on all trips that take them far from a doctor. Leaders responsible for others in remote areas should consider carrying injectable epinephrine. Epinephrine can be ruined by extremes of cold and heat. A prescription is required. **Consult your physician.** Once the epinephrine opens the airway and allows the patient to swallow, an antihistamine, preferably diphenhydramine, should be given immediately. The patient should be kept on the antihistamine during the evacuation to a hospital.

Asthma

Asthma is a recurring disease of the airway that causes swelling, increased mucus production, and spasms of the lower airway. Patients suffer moderate to severe respiratory difficulty during attacks. Air is often trapped in the lungs causing the patient to breath slowly with difficulty and a wheezing sound. Treatment includes calm encouragement of the patient to relax and breathe with control. Asthmatics should carry inhalers at all times, and extras on extended backcountry expeditions or trips to foreign countries. Assistance with the inhaler may be required. The medication in the inhaler must be sucked deep into the lungs to work. In extreme cases, injected epinephrine may open the blocked airway of an asthmatic. When the patient can swallow easily, drinking lots of water should be encouraged. Do **not** give the asthma patient antihistamines.

Diabetes

Patients with diabetes who have control of their disease with daily monitoring of their blood sugar, insulin injections, and diet are capable of every outdoor activity. On cold trips, insulin should carefully protected from freezing. Twice as much insulin, syringes, and batteries for the glucometer should be carried than would normally be needed, and it should not all be carried by the same person.

A patient with diabetes may experience the dangerous rapid onset of **hypoglycemia** (with low blood sugar, a **true emergency** characterized by an altered (confused) level of consciousness that leads quickly to great hunger, pale skin, and unconsciousness. The patient should eat or drink something sugary as soon as possible. If she or he is unconscious, sugar or sugary substances, e.g., the commercial product Glutose®, should be rubbed into the gums and under the tongue with the patient lying on his or her side. Untreated, death follows.

A patient with diabetes may also experience the slow onset of **hyperglycemia** (with high blood sugar) with accompanying great fatigue, great thirst, and the need to urinate. Untreated, high blood sugar leads to dehydration, a fruity odor on the breath, confusion, and coma. Treatment includes fluids and insulin. But insulin should **never** be injected except by a qualified physician. If unsure, give sugar—and evacuate the patient.

Heart Attack

Heart attack still leads to more deaths than any other cause in the United States. Patients complain of center-chest discomfort: crushing, squeezing pain or heavy pressure. Pain may radiate to shoulder, down the arm, into the jaw, predominantly on the left side. Nausea, sweating, and shortness of breath are common. Patients often deny the possibility that this could be a heart attack. In the backcountry, there is little to be done other than keeping the patient physically and emotional calm, in a position of comfort, and warm. Do not allow the patient to walk. If available, give the patient one-half a standard aspirin. Help needs to be sought. If the patient has been prescribed nitroglycerin, one pill should be placed under the tongue with the patient sitting down. Most physicians recommend a second pill if the first fails to work, and a third if the second fails to work. **Consult your physician.**

Hyperventilation Syndrome

Far from home, pain and/or fear often cause the patient to breathe faster and deeper than normal. This hyperventilation may lead to chest tightness, tingling or numbness in the hands, feet and/or face, and spasms in the hands and feet, which lead to more fear, which leads to more hyperventilation. The patient will either calm down or pass out. If he or she passes out, breathing may stop for what seems like a very long time. Except in rare circumstances, the patient will indeed start breathing again. (**Note:** If he or she doesn't, give a few mouth-to-mouth breaths.) Hyperventilating patients need to be calmed and encouraged to breathe normally. When calmness returns, then you can investigate the cause of the pain or fear.

Seizures

A great variety of causes can produce the uncontrollable rigid, jerky muscular movements of a seizure (or convulsion). Many people suffer seizure disorders and take drugs to prevent a seizure. The overstimulation of backcountry ventures has been known to encourage seizures, even in people taking preventive drugs. During a seizure, which normally lasts no more than two minutes, the patient needs protection from harmful objects, but the patient does **not** need restraint. Do **not** place anything in the patient's mouth. After the seizure, the patient will usually feel extreme fatigue and the need to sleep. Let the patient rest, preferably in a side position to maintain an open airway. Do not leave the patient alone. Check for injuries that may have occurred during the seizure. The

patient may require time and privacy to recover from some
of the common results of a seizure, such as incontinence.
Seizures for unknown reasons need a doctor's consultation.
Seizures for known reasons should initiate heart-to-heart
talks about the wisdom of continuing the trip.

20: Gender Specific Problems
For Women Only

Alterations in normal menstrual cycles are not unusual
for women in the outdoors. Unusual abdominal pain,
however, associated with abnormal vaginal bleeding should
be reported to a physician as soon as possible. Pelvic pain
with fever and chills, nausea and vomiting, and perhaps a
watery, foul-smelling vaginal discharge also requires a
physician's attention.

Symptoms of **vaginal infection** may include excessive or
malodorous vaginal discharge with redness, itching and,
perhaps, a burning sensation during urination. Women
with a history of vaginal infections should carry appropriate
medications: Gyne-Lotrimin® or Monistat®. If the medications don't provide relief within 48 hours, the patient
should see a doctor. In extreme circumstances, the patient
may consider a douche with plain disinfected water or with
a solution of two tablespoons of vinegar in a liter of warm
disinfected water. A douche can also be made from two
tablespoons of povidone-iodine solution in a liter of water.

Urinary tract infections cause increased frequency and urgency of urination, often with a burning sensation on urination. Low abdominal pain is common. Blood or pus may appear in the urine. The patient should drink lots of water, and avoid sugary foods and foods that irritate the bladder, e.g., caffeine, alcohol, peppery foods. The perineal area should be washed daily with water and mild soap. On extended trips, women should consider carrying an antibiotic for UTI. Ciprofloxacin (sold as Cipro®) is often prescribed. **Consult your physician.** (*Note:* Men are not immune to UTI.)

For Men Only

Epididymitis, an inflammation of the epididymis, tends to come on slowly, possibly with a fever, and a red, swollen, painful scrotum. The patient suffers, and the only immediate relief is found in rest, support for the scrotum, e.g., jockstrap, or improvised support from a triangular bandage, and painkillers. Antibiotics are necessary. Evacuate the patient to a physician.

Torsion of the Testis is a twisting of the testis within the scrotum. Pain may come on suddenly or slowly. Scrotum is red, swollen, and painful. The lack of blood supply means death for the testis in about 24 hours. Evacuate the patient. Cool compresses and painkillers provide some relief. A jockstrap, or improvised support, may give some more relief and may increase blood flow to the testis. If the evacuation will be long, attempt to rotate the painful testis into a normal position. Since most testicles rotate "inward," a gentle rotation "outward" may give immediate and blessed relief. The patient may wish to make the rotation himself. If it doesn't work, perhaps the testicle rotated in the opposite direction, so rotate the testicle two turns in the opposite direction. If you fail, the patient is no worse off than before the attempt was made.

21: Common Simple Problems

Blisters

Those fluid-filled bubbles are mild burns caused by friction. Friction produces a separation of the tough outer layer of skin from the sensitive inner layer. Only where skin is hardened is it thick enough for this to happen—heels, toes, soles, palms. Loose skin just wears away with friction, leaving an abrasion. Blisters range from unpleasant to terribly debilitating. But they are not a serious problem unless they become infected.

What should you do? Blisters feel better when the bubble is deflated, and controlled draining is far better than having them rupture inside a dirty sock. Clean around the site thoroughly. Sterilize the point of a needle or knife, or use a sterile scalpel to open the blister. Massage the fluid out. Leaving the roof of the blister intact will make it feel better and heal faster. If the roof has been rubbed away, treat the wound as you would any other *(see Wound*

Management). Apply a dressing that limits friction: 2nd Skin®, or a moleskin "donut" (a piece of moleskin with a hole cut in the center) filled with ointment, or ointment and a gauze pad over the blister. Whatever you put over the drained blister requires tape or moleskin strips to hold it in place.

Blisters can be prevented by 1) wearing boots or shoes that fit and are broken in, 2) wearing a thin inner sock under a thicker outer sock, 3) treating "hot spots" with moleskin, 2nd Skin®, tape, or tincture of benzoin compound **before** they become blisters, and 4) taking off your boots to let your feet dry when you take a break from hiking.

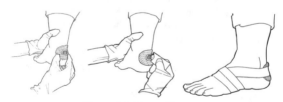

Figure 20: Blister Treatment

Diarrhea

The backcountry is home to a multitude of diarrhea-causing life forms: protozoa, bacteria, viruses. They will produce, generally speaking, one of two kinds of diarrhea:

1) **Non-invasive diarrhea**, with microbial colonies on upper small intestine walls, leading to abdominal cramping, nausea, vomiting, and massive amounts of water, filled with salt and potassium, rushing out of the bowels. 2) **Invasive diarrhea**, sometimes called dysentery, with bacteria attacking the lower small intestine and colon, causing inflammation, bloody bowel movements, fever, abdominal cramping, and painful release of loose stools.

Whatever the cause, dehydration is the immediate problem with diarrhea. Mild diarrhea can be treated with water or diluted fruit juices or diluted sports drinks. Persistent diarrhea requires more aggressive replacement of electrolytes lost in the stool. Oral rehydration solutions are best for treating serious diarrhea. You can get by, usually, adding one tsp. salt and eight tsp. sugar to a liter of water. The patient should drink about one-fourth of this solution every hour, along with all the water he or she will tolerate. Rice, grains, bananas, potatoes are OK to eat. Fats, dairy products, caffeine and alcohol should be avoided.

Over-the-counter medications for watery diarrhea are available. Prescription medications include Lomotil®. Dysentery should be treated with antibiotics, not medicinal plugs. **Consult your physician concerning prescription drugs.**

Dehydration

Water is easily and quickly lost from the body in the outdoors through sweating, urination, defecation, breathing, and diarrhea. Even mild dehydration causes loss of energy, loss of mental acuity, and loss of fun. Mild dehydration shows up as thirst, dry mouth and dark urine. Moderate dehydration adds very dry mouth, reduction of the amount of dark urine, a rapid weak pulse, and remarkable dizziness when the patient stands up. Severe dehydration very very dry mouth, lack of urine, and shock. Treatment of dehydration is explained above (see Diarrhea). Prevention is this: Drink lots of fluid, water or diluted sports drinks. Drink a half-liter every morning. Drink a quarter-liter every 15 to 20 minutes during periods of exercise. Drink enough to keep your urine clear.

Dental Problems

Where a filling has fallen out or a cavity has developed, pain usually first occurs when cold, food or your tongue hits the spot. After rinsing the area clean, a drop of oil of cloves (eugenol) will ease the pain. A temporary filling is the best treatment until a dentist can be found. Cavit® is the easiest to use and best temporary filling material. Just fill the hole with Cavit®, bit to align with the teeth above, and wait till it hardens. A temporary filling can be made from mixing zinc oxide powder and eugenol. To improvise, fill the cavity with candle wax, ski wax or sugarless gum. Temporary filling material can also be used to hold a dislodged crown back in place.

If a tooth is knocked out, there is a small chance it can be salvaged if you can get it back it the hole from whence it came. After rinsing the tooth off (do **not** scrub it), press it gently back in. If it won't go back in, at least save it until you find a dentist. Same goes for a broken off piece of tooth.

When a broken tooth exposes the pulp, pain can be extreme. A small piece of aspirin placed directly on the exposed pulp causes a burning pain but "cauterizes" the pulp, putting an end to the patient's distress for a while. **Never** put aspirin on the gum next to an aching tooth. Acid in aspirin will burn the gum. Swallow the aspirin, or another painkiller, if you need further relief.

Any bleeding inside the mouth can be given direct pressure with a gauze pad held in place with your finger or bitten in place with your teeth. A moistened non-herbal tea bag can be used instead of gauze—the tannic acid in tea initiates clotting. Avoid irritating a wound in the mouth: no smoking, no chewing on the "bad" side, no hot foods, no sucking on the wound.

An infected tooth is indicated by a lot of swelling in the gum and cheek near the tooth. Discoloration may be visible. This tooth needs a dentist as soon as possible. Cold packs on the cheek may give some relief. If evacuation is delayed, have the patient rinse her mouth several times a day with warm, salty water. It would be best to start the patient on an oral antibiotic. **Consult your physician** concerning antibiotics for tooth infection.

And consult your dentist at least one month prior to an extended backcountry trip or a journey to a foreign country in order to have potential problems identified and treated. Routine oral hygiene will prevent most trip-ruining dental problems: floss once a day, and brush twice a day with a soft-bristled toothbrush.

Ear Problems

Don't poke anything in your ear smaller than your elbow. If something is lodged in the ear, such as a small insect, try flushing it out with alcohol or water. Outer ear infections, or "swimmer's ear," hurt more when you pull on the earlobe. Flush the ear daily with dilute vinegar or alcohol. If pain persists, find a doctor. Middle ear infections do not increase in pain when the earlobe is tugged and are often accompanied with vertigo. These infections require antibiotic treatment—see a doctor.

Eye Problems

If the patient complains of something in the eye, look closely and try to identify the object. If it's lodged, leave it alone and find a doctor. If it's large and lodged, protect the object to prevent it being bumped, and carry the patient out sitting at approximately a 45-degree angle. If it's small and loose, flush it out or dab it out with a soft cloth. Once loose objects are removed, the patient may complain that it still feels like something is there. The eye is probably scratched—typically not serious, but the eye will heal faster if it's patched shut for 24 hours. A "black eye" is typically non-serious and self-limiting, but beware of injuries that produce visible cuts or any disturbance in vision—reasons to find a doctor. Swollen, red, itchy eyes with a colorful discharge are almost always infected. After flushing the eye with disinfected water, small amounts of antibiotic ointment may be placed in the eye several times a day. Ointments made for the eye are best. If the problem persists, it should be seen by a physician.

Fishhook Removal

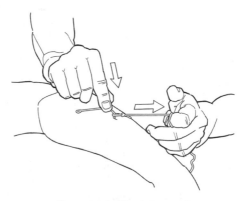

Figure 21: Fishhook Removal

The **string-pull technique** requires a loop of string: Place the loop around the curve of the hook, push down on the hook to loosen the barb, yank the loop—the hook pops out. The **push-through-and-snip technique** requires pushing the embedded hook out through the skin, snipping off the barb, and backing the hook out. If it is large and deeply imbedded hook, you will have to slice delicately with a sharp edge to loosen the hook prior to removal.

Headache

A common outdoor complaint, headaches have three general causes: 1) dehydration, 2) muscular tension, and 3) a vascular disorder. Most headaches respond to rest, hydration, massage and over-the-counter painkillers, e.g., ibuprofen. Beware of the headache that comes on suddenly, is unrelieved by rest and medication, and is not like any other headache you've ever had. Find a doctor.

Nosebleed

Lean the patient forward and pinch the meaty part of the nose firmly shut. Hold it for 10 to 15 minutes. If bleeding persists, a squirt of a nose spray, such as Afrin®, may help stop the bleeding. If the bleeding still persists, pack the nostrils gently with gauze soaked with antibiotic ointment or a spray such as Afrin®. It is possible for noses to bleed from the back, and blood runs down the throat. These posterior nosebleeds need a physician's attention.

Snowblindness

Six to twelve hours after overexposure to the sun's radiation, the patient complains of pain and swelling in the eye with a feeling like an "eye full of sand." The cornea of the eye has been sunburned. Sunburned eyes are usually very sensitive to light. Rinses with cool water will clean the eye and ease the pain. Cool compresses may be applied for pain. A small amount of antibiotic ointment may be applied several times a day for two to three days. Ointments made for the eye are best. The patient's eyes may need to be covered for 24 hours. Snowblindness almost always resolves harmlessly in 24 to 48 hours. Prolonged discomfort is reason to see a physician. The problem can be prevented by wearing sunglasses that block UV radiation. On snow or water, sunglasses should fit well and have side-shields to block reflected UV light.

Splinters

Splinters should be removed as soon as possible. If the end is visible, grasp it with tweezers and pull it gently out. If the end is buried, probe with your fingers until you find the orientation of the splinter, and push it toward the wound until the end is graspable. With deeply buried splinters, you may need to cut superficially with a sterile scalpel to expose the embedded object. Clean and dress any resulting wounds.

Sunburn

The immediate response to overexposure to ultraviolet light is burned skin. Prolonged exposure, over years, leads to premature skin aging and degenerative skin disorders such as cancer. First aid for sunburn includes cooling the skin, applying a moisturizer, ibuprofen for pain and inflammation, and staying out of direct sunlight. If blisters form, a doctor should be consulted. Prevention of sunburn includes hats with brims and tightly-woven clothing, sunblocks such as zinc oxide, and sunscreens with a high sun protection factor—SPF 15 or more. Be aware: You can burn on cloudy days, sunlight is most harmful between the hours of 10AM and 3PM, and large amounts of UV light are reflected by snow and water.

Water Disinfection

A lot of gastrointestinal distress can be avoided at home and abroad if you disinfect all drinking water. There are three methods that work:

Boiling kills organisms that make people sick. In fact, the time it takes water to reach the boiling point, even at high altitudes, kills organisms. So by the time water has reached the point of boiling, it is safe to drink.

Filters differ greatly in their ability to disinfect water. Some filter out only protozoa, such as Giardia and Cryptosporidium. Some filter out protozoa and bacteria.

None filter out viruses, but some have an iodine-resin on the filter that may kill viruses. Choose carefully.

Chemicals can be added to water to kill harmful organisms. Iodine and chlorine are safest and most effective, but no chemical guarantees water safe from Cryptosporidium. In most cases, iodine is the preferred chemical because it stores better and reacts less with organic compounds in water. Iodine is commercially available in several forms including tablets such as Potable Aqua® and crystals. If you have povidone-iodine solution in your first aid kit, it can be used to disinfect water. The solution is best measured with a dropper. Eight (8) drops of povidone-iodine solution in warm clear water, and a 15-minute wait will give you a safe drink. In cold clear water, double the drops and double the wait (16 drops for 30 minutes). In cloudy water, double the drops and triple the wait.

22: First Aid for Children

When hiking into remote geographical locations with children, your medical knowledge and your first aid kit should be adapted to meet their special smaller bodies. Although specific needs may differ from trip to trip depending on such variables as the ages of the children, the length of the trip, the time of year of the trip, and any pre-existing medical conditions, some medical advice is useful for all younger ages.

Kids and Heat

Children gain core heat faster than adults. Little human cooling systems work fine, mostly, but they sometimes need encouragement. The younger the child the less developed their internal heat regulating system, and the larger their surface area for heat dissipation in relation to their body mass.

Allow your children time to acclimatize to heat. It will take them longer than it will take you. Early in the hot season, or early into a trip to an area hotter than your child is used to, go easy for the first few days, and increase the activity level progressively. The human body becomes increasingly able to withstand the heat.

Encourage your child to drink lots of water. And don't be surprised if they claim a lack of thirst. Children feel the need to drink less readily than adults. Thirst is a sign that the body has already entered the early stages of dehydration. The old proverb advising "you can't drink too much water" is technically false but practically true (*see Hyponatremia*). Water loss from your child can be significant during one hour of activity in a warm climate. If you find it difficult to get kids to drink plain water, add enough powdered flavoring to make the water less boring, but not enough to make it a syrup.

Kids and Diarrhea

Children dehydrate faster than adults, and fluid loss, especially via diarrhea, can be devastating. One of the best and earliest signs of dehydration is urine color: Clear indicates a well-hydrated child (or adult) and dark yellow indicates poor hydration. As dehydration grows worse, watch for headache, unusual fatigue, loss of appetite, nausea, and other complaints that make you think flu. One of the later signs of serious dehydration in a child is restlessness and unusual loss of interest in whatever's going on around them.

For treating diarrhea, carry a mild anti-diarrheal medication in your first aid kit. Children should continue to eat during episodes of diarrhea. Avoid milk for a day. Infants do well on rice cereal, apple sauce, and bananas for a day or two. Older children may eat plain dry toast, plain crackers, plain chicken soup, and other bland foods. After the first couple of days, yogurt helps to repopulate the bowels with healthy bacteria.

Kids and Dehydration

For treating dehydration, whether from diarrhea, vomiting, or heat, use oral rehydration salts (ORS) instead of plain water. ORS replaces essential salts and contains a little sugar for energy. You can buy ORS or make your own rehydration solution by adding one teaspoon of sugar and a pinch of salt to one quart of water. Do not use salt tablets.

Kids and Sunshine

The sun is worse on kids than it is on adults, even though the damage may not show up for thirty years. Eighty percent of skin damage from the sun (including skin cancers) happens in the first couple of decades of life.

Children sunburn more easily than adults. Children should wear clothing woven tight enough to protect their skin from ultraviolet (UV) light, and hats with a brim to protect their faces, and sunscreen on unprotected skin. Ultraviolet A and B damage skin, and the sunscreen should protect against both. Assume the SPF (Sun Protection Factor) is not as good as it claims and use a higher number. Sunscreens should be applied in a uniform coat over all exposed areas. If your trip involves swimming, use a waterproof sunscreen, and reapply it often. A few inches of water will not protect your child's skin from sunburn. Once a pleasant suntan is established, the screen should still be used. Tans prevent burning but offer little protection from the harmful effects of the sun.

Keep children under one year out of the sun as much as possible, and apply sunscreens to their sensitive skin only when absolutely necessary. Test the screen on a small portion of skin, about the size of your hand, first to see if the child will react. If they do react, try a different brand. For young children, use a screen prepared as a milky lotion or cream, and avoid the upper and lower eyelids where the screen might be rubbed involuntarily into the eye. Never use baby oil in the sun. Encourage children to wear sunglasses in order to reduce the chance of cataracts later in life, and to protect their sensitive eyelids.

If your child gets a sunburn, start treatment as soon as possible. Cool compresses may reduce the pain and limit the depth of the burn. Moisturizing lotions should be applied to skin. Acetaminophen may be given for pain. Drinking lots of water is important in the treatment of sunburn.

Kids and Insects

Children have more trouble than adults, usually, resisting the temptation to scratch itchy bites. Because they are also typically less hygienic than adults, scratches on children have a higher rate of infection. Sting wipes may be used immediately to reduce the temptation to scratch. Hydrocortisone cream will reduce the itch of more established bites. To improvise an anti-itch medication, you may use a slurry of baking soda or meat tenderizer. Bites that are scratched open should be washed with soap and water, and covered with an adhesive strip dressing.

For prevention, insect repellent should be used regularly. DEET, a common repelling ingredient, should not be used in a high concentration. For children, the lower the concentration the better. Keep the repellent off children's hands, and you'll reduce the chance they'll rub it into their eyes or, even worse, suck it off their fingers. You can avoid DEET by choosing products made with natural repellents, such as Repel Lemon Eucalyptus®.

Kids and Poisons

Campsites should be checked closely in order to identify the presence of poison oak, sumac, or ivy. Children should be made aware of, and taught how to identify and avoid, all poisonous plants. If contact is suspected, all skin that may have contacted the poisonous plant should be washed immediately with soft soap and cool water. Clothing, including shoes, that may have contacted the poisonous plant should be cleaned thoroughly. If the itch, redness and fluid-filled bumps of a reaction to the plants develop on skin, hydrocortisone cream or calamine lotion may be used to treat the symptoms. Only time will bring healing.

Small children make up the great majority of ingested poison patients. In a suspected poisoning, you may consider inducing vomiting as soon as possible. The child should first be given water to drink—at least eight ounces. Then gently stimulate the gag reflex with your finger. Do not induce vomiting in children who 1) are having seizures, 2) are lethargic or in danger of further loss of consciousness, 3) have already vomited, 4) have ingested a corrosive substance (which usually produces burns on the lips on in the mouth), or 5) have ingested a petroleum product. If the child has ingested a poison, he or she should be evacuated to a medical facility as soon as possible, even if vomiting has occurred. Prevent poisoning by clearly identifying to the child anything in the environment that should be avoided, and keeping all dangerous substances out of reach.

Kids and Medications

Children aged five and under usually can't swallow pills. Carry chewable tablets. For children too little to chew, the tablets can be crushed and added to food. Some children's medications are available in liquid form, less desirable for backcountry trips, but it might be your best choice. For pain and/or fever, acetaminophen and/or ibuprofen are typically recommended. You may wish to carry an antihistamine. **Consult your physician.**

Kids Get Lost

To help prevent children from wandering off indiscreetly into the wild places, set strict boundaries around campsites. Supply children with whistles and a code: Three blows means "help"...two blows means "we hear you!" Encourage children to hug-a-tree (stay put) if they get lost.

Kids and Ouchies

Little people get scraped and cut and blistered just like big people, but they sometimes make less than perfect patients. To encourage kid cooperation, carry kid-oriented wound management products, e.g., adhesive strips with cartoon characters on them.

23: Advice to International Travelers

Malaria

Malaria ranks as a leading cause of death on this planet. Once thought to result from breathing "swamp gas," the moist fumes rising from wet areas, malaria literally means "bad air." But all four species of the parasite that cause the disease get into human blood only from the bite of the female *Anopheles* mosquito. Malaria is the greatest health risk to US travelers to any region where the disease exists.

Your "ounce of prevention" should include everything possible to avoid mosquito bites: Clothing thick enough to prevent 'skeeter nose penetration, insecticide, e.g., permethrin, on your clothes. Repellents containing N, N-diethyl-meta-toluamide (a.k.a. N, N-diethyl-3-methylbenzamide)—better known as DEET—on exposed skin. (**Note:** DEET should be used strictly in accordance with directions on the label and washed off skin as soon as exposure to mosquitoes has ended.) Non-DEET repellents such as Repel Lemon Eucalyptus®. Netting to sleep under. Avoidance of mosquito prime time—they are primarily dusk and nocturnal feeders. This, unfortunately, seldom meets all your prevention needs, and accidental exposure to an infected mosquito is virtually guaranteed in high-risk areas.

So, to be as safe as possible, you'll have to resort to chemical prophylaxis. The drug of choice for prevention of malaria has long been chloroquine (and it still is in many regions of the world), but some parasites have developed a resistance to it. In March, 1990, the Centers for Disease Control (CDC) made mefloquine the officially approved drug in chloroquine-resistant areas. **Consult your physician.** Although normal side-effects with mefloquine are minimal, some people—people with high blood pressure or heart problems—should take the drug only under careful physician supervision. Controversy exists concerning the use of mefloquine by children and pregnant women.

Food and Water

Amoebic dysentery, diarrheal diseases, and parasitic worms are associated with poor choice of water and food in many countries. Disinfect all water before drinking or brushing your teeth or mixing your cocktails. Avoid milk, butter, and other dairy products. Watch bottled drinks being uncapped before you accept one. Make sure all food is well-cooked and served hot. Fruits with intact skins are safe if peeled shortly before consumption. Don't go swimming in backcountry lakes, ponds and streams where there is any chance of acquiring the fluke that causes schistosomiasis.

Vaccinations

Don't leave home without checking with your
physician and/or the Centers for Disease Control (CDC)
about what vaccinations to get and other precautions to
take before entering the foreign countries on your itinerary.
Allow six to eight weeks to make sure to have time to get
everything done that they recommend. Current
recommendations for US travelers issued by the CDC are
found in *Health Information for International Travel*
(published annually). The publication contains vaccination
and certification requirements on a country-by-country
basis. It also has the US Public Health Service
recommendations for difficult immunization questions,
such as immunization of infants, breast feeding and
pregnant women, and specific recommendations for
vaccination and prophylaxis for each of a wide variety of
disorders. It also contains a discussion of specific potential
health hazards worldwide by geographic region. The
information in this book is updated in the biweekly
Summary of Health Information for International Travel. Both
the book and updates can be obtained from the
Superintendent of Documents, US Government Printing
Office, Washington, DC 20402. They are also carried by
many major libraries, nearly all health departments and
travelers' clinics.

In general, all travelers should make sure their
childhood immunizations are up to date, immunizations

that include polio, measles, mumps, diphtheria, and whooping cough. All travelers should be assured of their tetanus immunity, and should consider acquiring immunity to hepatitis A.

Sources of Information

Questions about special health considerations and new developments in things-to-watch-out-for will be answered on the CDC's 24-hour **International Traveler's Hotline:** (877) FYI-TRIP. Or go to www.cdc.gov.

You might also consider packing the *International Association for Medical Assistance to Traveler's* (IAMAT) list of worldwide English-speaking physicians. The list is free of charge: IAMAT, 417 Center Street, Lewiston, NY 14092; (716) 754-4883.

An alternative source of information is the publication, *Vaccination Certificate Requirements and Health Advice for International Travelers*, published yearly by the World Health Organization, Geneva, Switzerland. It is less specific and less comprehensive than the CDC publication.

Refer also to the definitive effort by William W. Forgey, MD: *Travelers' Medical Resource*, The Globe Pequot Press, P. O. Box 480, Guilford, CT 06437; (800) 962-0973.

Medical Kits

All international travelers should carry their own first aid kit, especially trekkers who end up well away from

medical assistance of any sort. Your physician will probably
be willing to help you put together the hard-to-find items
you'll want to have along. The kit should include a brief
written personal medical history including allergies and
recent illnesses, and any prescription drugs you are
personally using with written directions for their use
and—in case some border guard thinks you're a smuggler—
a copy of the prescription. Note: If you use or think you'll
need an injected drug, carry your own sterile syringes. It is
not safe to rely on the sterility of needles in many countries.
Carry painkillers, antacids, antihistamines, anti-diarrhea
medications, insect repellent, sunscreen, a means to
disinfect water, wound management materials including
ointment, gauze, tape and other bandages, and a few basic
splinting materials. Remember a first aid kit functions only
at the level of the person using it. If you really want to take
of yourself and others in remote settings, pack some
training into your brain.

24: Non-Prescription Drugs

   Note: When using these, or any medications, follow
the directions on the label and/or your physician's
advice. Children and pregnant women should not take
medications without first consulting a physician.

Acetaminophen (e.g., Tylenol®):

For relief of pain of headache, cold and flu discomfort, minor muscle and joint discomfort, and menstrual cramps. For reduction of fever. Especially useful for those who are allergic to aspirin or aspirin-containing products. Does <u>not</u> work as an anti-inflammatory.

Antacid Tablets (e.g., Mylanta®, Magnacal®):

For symptomatic relief of heartburn, acid indigestion, sour stomach, and other conditions related to an upset stomach. Mylanta® helps relieve intestinal gas problems.

Antibiotic Ointment:

Contains ingredients that may help prevention of infection in minor wounds, encourages healing of wounds, works as a lubricant, some relief for itching.

Antihistamine (e.g., diphenhydramine):

For the temporary relief of respiratory allergy symptoms and cold symptoms. Helps relieve the itching of allergic skin reactions. May be used as a mild sedative. Critical in the treatment of anaphylaxis.

Aspirin:

Same uses as acetaminophen but **does** work as an anti-inflammatory. Can be used to "cauterize" exposed tooth pulp. May be helpful during heart attacks. Not to be given to children. Many people are allergic to aspirin.

Decongestant Spray (e.g., Afrin® Nasal Spray):
For relief of nasal congestion that accompanies cold and allergies. May be useful to help stop nosebleed. May be useful to relieve sinus "squeeze" from diving.

Decongestant Tablet (e.g., Dristan®, Fedrin®):
For symptomatic relief of sinus headache pain and pressure caused by sinus congestion. A multi-purpose cold medicine.

Diarrhea Medication (e.g., Imodium®, Diarrest®):
For use in the control of diarrhea.

Electrolytes (tablets or solution):
For use in replacing electrolytes lost due to prolonged diarrhea, sweating, etc. Can be used as an adjunct in preventing heat exhaustion and muscle cramps due to excessive sweating.

Fungus Treatment Cream (e.g., Tinactin®):
For treatment of superficial skin fungi such as ringworm, jock itch, and athlete's foot.

Hydrocortisone Cream:
May provide relief of pain and itching of poison ivy, poison oak, poison oak, insect bites, and other allergic skin reactions. May help dry up oozing rash of allergic skin reactions.

Ibuprofen (e.g., Advil®):

For symptomatic relief of pain associated with headache, colds, flu, frostbite, toothache, arthritis, burns, and menstrual cramps. For pain of inflammation associated muscle and joint injury and overuse. Helps reduce a fever.

Pepto-Bismol®:

For use in the control of diarrhea, nausea and upset stomach. May help prevent "traveler's diarrhea." Not to be taken by the aspirin-allergic.

25: Prescription Drugs

Note: Consult a physician before choosing to carry or use any prescription medication. Carry written instructions concerning indications for use, doses, and contraindications. Know if you are allergic to any drugs before taking them. Pregnant women and children should use no drugs without a physician's advice.

DRUG	COMMENTS	DOSAGE
Analgesics (Painkillers)		
Percocet®	For severe pain. Narcotic. Do not stay in the back country.	One tablet every four to eight hours.

DRUG	COMMENTS	DOSAGE
Tylenol®#3	For moderate to severe pain. Also good for diarrhea and coughs. Contains codeine, a narcotic.	One or two tablets every four to six hours.
Vicodin®	For moderate to severe pain	One or two tablets every four to six hours
Antibiotics		
Cephalexin (e.g., Keflex®)	For skin, bone, pneumonia and urinary tract infections. ***Beware if penicillin allergy exists.***	250 to 500mg every six hours.
Ciprofloxacin (Cipro®)	Best for infectious diarrheas. Okay for bone and urinary tract infections. ***Not for children***	500mg every 12 hours

Drug	Comments	Dosage
Erythromycin	For sinus, pulmonary, ear, eye, respiratory and soft tissue infections. Okay if penicillin allergy exists.	250 to 500mg every six hours. Take with food.
Anti-Diarrheal		
Lomotil®	For severe diarrhea.	Two tablets with each loose stool up to 8 tablets per day
Anti-Emetic (for vomiting)		
Phenergan®	For severe nausea and vomiting.	One 25 mg suppository every four hours as needed.
Anti-Allergy		
Epinephrine (Ana-Kit® or Epi-Pen®)	For severe allergic reactions, inject the pre-measured doses of 0.3cc.	

DRUG	COMMENTS	DOSAGE
Altitude Illness		
Acetazolamide (Diamox®)	For altitude illness. To be used **with** descent. May prevent illness when taken prophylactically.	125mg two times per day.
Dexamethasone (Decadron®)	For High Altitude Cerebral Edema. Steroid. To be used **with** descent.	8mg to start, 4mg every six hours during evacuation.
Anti-Vertigo (for motion sickness)		
Meclizine (e.g. Antivert®)	For motion sickness.	25–100mg daily started at least one hour prior to motion.

About the Author

Buck Tilton's dynamic personality and great concern for the outdoor enthusiast have led him to become known worldwide as a respected instructor of wilderness medicine and an expert in extended care. He is co-founder of the Wilderness Medicine Institute of the National Outdoor Leadership School, P.O. Box 9, Pitkin, Colorado 81241. He has authored or coauthored 23 books including *The Wilderness First Responder, Medicine for the Backcountry 3rd Edition, Basic Essentials of Rescue from the Backcountry, Basic Essentials of Avalanche Safety,* and *Camping Healthy.* In addition to many writing and teaching responsibilities, Buck serves as consultant to WPC Brands, Inc., Jackson, WI.